COLUMBIA COLLEGE
616.951R579S   C1   V0

THE SEXUALLY TRANSMITTED DISEASES$ JE

3 2711 00003 7742

Y0-EAJ-619

616.951 R579s

Rinear, Charles E., 1949-

APR '98

ENTERED APR 0 7 1992

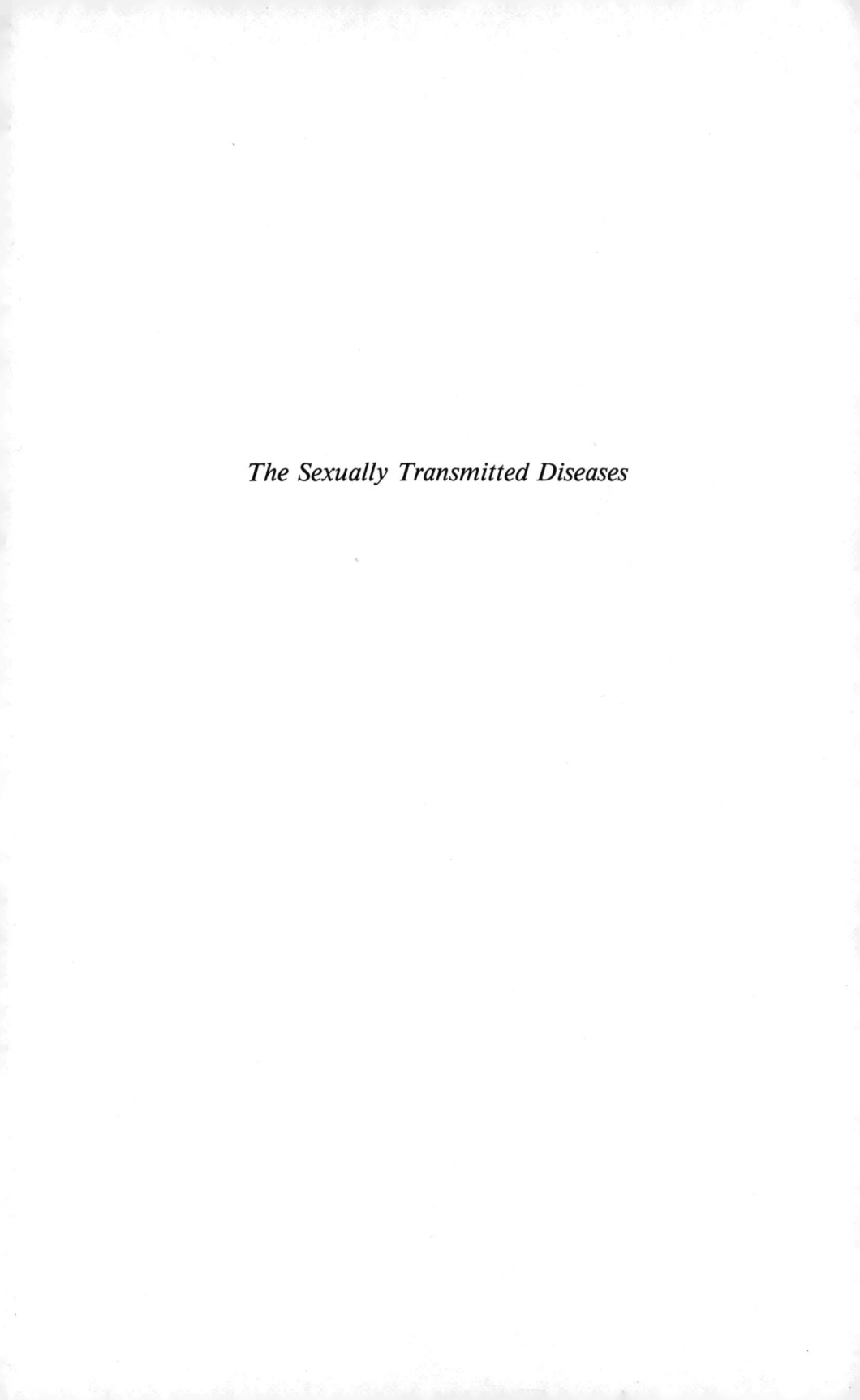

The Sexually Transmitted Diseases

The Sexually Transmitted Diseases

Charles E. Rinear

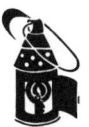

McFarland & Company, Inc., Publishers
Jefferson, North Carolina, and London

```
616.951 R579s

Rinear, Charles E., 1949-

The sexually transmitted
 diseases
```

Library of Congress Cataloguing-in-Publication Data

Rinear, Charles E., 1949–
  The sexually transmitted diseases.

  Includes references.
  Includes index.
  1. Venereal diseases.   I. Title. [DNLM:
  1. Venereal Diseases.   WC 140 R579s]
  RC200.R56   1986   616.95′1   85-14964

ISBN 0-89950-185-0 (acid-free natural paper)

© 1986 Charles E. Rinear. All rights reserved.

Printed in the United States of America.

McFarland   Box 611   Jefferson NC 28640

This book is respectfully dedicated
to all people attempting to solve the problem
of STDs throughout the world.

Table of Contents

Acknowledgments   ix
Introduction   1

1. Acquired Immune Deficiency Syndrome (AIDS)   5
2. Chancroid   28
3. Condylomata Acuminata   32
4. Ctyomegalovirus Infection (CMV)   36
5. Enteric Infections   39
    Amebiasis   40
    Cryptosporidiosis   44
    Giardiasis   44
    Shigellosis   47
6. Gonococcal Disease   50
    Gonorrhea of Columnar and Transitional Epithelium   50
    Gonococcal Vulvovaginitis of Female Children   60
    Gonococcal Ophthalmia Neonatorum   62
    Metastatic Gonorrhea or Disseminated
      Gonococcal Infections (DGI)   65
    Penicillinase-Producing Neisseria Gonorrhoeae   90
7. Granuloma Inguinale   96
8. Group B Hemolytic Streptococcal Infections   100
9. Herpes Progenitalis   104
10. Lymphogranuloma Venereum   116
11. Molluscum Contagiosum   120
12. Nonspecific Nongonococcal Urethritis   123
13. Pediculosis Pubis (Crabs)   130
14. Pinta   134
15. Reiter's Syndrome   137
16. Scabies   140
17. Urinary Tract Infections   143
18. Vaginitis   148
    Candidiasis   148

      Gardnerella Vaginale Vaginitis   153
      Nonspecific Vaginitis   156
      Trichomoniasis   156
19. Venereal Syphilis   162
20. Viral Hepatitis Infections   189
21. Yaws   193
22. Toward the Prevention and Control of Sexually Transmitted Diseases   196

References   203
Index   209

Acknowledgments

The author gratefully acknowledges the following individuals who have contributed to his knowledge of public health as it relates to sexually transmitted diseases:

James Hoxie, M.D., cancer specialist and AIDS researcher, the hospital of the University of Pennsylvania.

Jerome Goldstein, M.D., P.C., dermatologist in private practice and adjunct professor of Medicine at the Hahnamann University Medical Center.

Leon Bacchues, Psy.D., psychologist with the Philadelphia AIDS Task Force.

Eileen Rinear, R.N., Ph.D., director of community health education, North Penn Hospital; adjunct professor of Health Education at Temple University.

Frank H. Jenne, Ph.D., M.P.H., professor of Health Education at Temple University.

Marvin R. Levy, Ed.D., M.P.H., professor of Health Education at Temple University.

Walter H. Greene, Ed.D., professor of Health Education at Temple University.

Mary Anne Smith, M.D., specialist in internal medicine in private practice.

Neil E. Gallagher, Ph.D., professor and chairperson, the Department of Health Science at Towson State University.

Geraldine Baird, D.O., specialist in internal medicine in private practice.

Introduction

The sexually transmitted diseases (STDs) are those primarily acquired by sexual contact.[1,2] Medical authorities conservatively estimate that at least 30 sexually transmitted diseases exist and that at least 10 million Americans are affected by such diseases within the United States alone each year.[3,4] Formerly known as "venereal diseases," or "V.D.," sexually transmitted diseases are ordinarily found only in humans.[5,6]

The 30 major forms of sexually transmissible disease include the traditional five, gonorrhea, venereal syphilis, chancroid, granuloma inguinale, and lymphogranuloma venereum, along with 25 others, which have been added to what appears to be an ever-increasing and alarming list.[7,8,9] This list presently includes the following diseases:[9]

*Acquired Immunodeficiency
  Syndrome
Chancroid
Condylomata Acuminata
Cytomegalovirus Infections
Enteric Infections (four major
  types)
Gonococcal Disease (four major
  types)
Granuloma Inguinale
Group B Hemolytic Streptococcal
  Infections
Herpes Progenitalis*

*Lymphogranuloma Venereum
Molluscum Contagiosum
Nonspecific Nongonococcal
  Urethritis
Pediculosis Pubis
Pinta
Reiter's Syndrome
Scabies
Urinary Tract Infections
Vaginitis (four major types)
Veneral Syphilis
Viral Hepatitis Infections
Yaws*

It should be emphasized that medical and public health authorities sometimes disagree on what constitutes a sexually transmitted disease along with how to classify and otherwise conceptualize these diseases. Whatever one's classification system, sexually transmitted diseases clearly represent one of the most alarming and threatening health problems of all times.[13,14] During World War II when penicillin treatment was initiated, it was predicted that the two major venereal diseases (gonorrhea and syphilis) would be eradicated.[1,10] However, with a worldwide estimated prevalence of 150 million cases of gonorrhea along with one million reported cases of gonorrhea and 22,000 reported cases of venereal syphilis within the United States alone each year (a new case of gonorrhea or syphilis every 14 seconds), this hardly appears to be the case.[12,13,14]

The Size of the Problem

The incidence and prevalence of sexually transmitted diseases had been climbing steadily in epidemic proportions until 1978, when medical and public health authorities reported the first decline in the incidence and prevalence of gonorrhea and syphilis within 20 years.[13] However, the incidence and prevalence of the other STDs such as nongonococcal urethritis, herpes progenitalis, and acquired immune deficiency syndrome (AIDS) appear to be skyrocketing.[9,13,14] Furthermore, it must be fully appreciated that the true incidence and prevalence of these diseases (in contrast to *reported cases*) is estimated by some medical and public authorities to be three to four times higher than the officially reported rates.[13] In actuality, there may be three to four million cases of gonorrhea in the United States along with 80,000 cases of syphilis. There are perhaps some 10 million cases of herpes infection in the U.S. with some 300,000 new infections per year, if statistics from the Herpes Resource Center are accurate.[4,11,13,14] Depending upon one's source and whether reported or estimated cases are included, these statistics vary greatly; for example, the Pennsylvania Department of Health notes that there are perhaps some five million cases of herpes infection within the U.S.[11]

Sexually transmitted diseases affect both sexes, all ages, all races, all social classes, and people from every educational and occupational background. However, some authorities believe that perhaps some 75 percent of all STDs affect individuals 15 to 30 years of age and that perhaps 50 to 75 percent of syphilis cases involve gay men.[13] Some authorities believe that at least one in every 50 teenagers will contract gonorrhea and that as many as half of all young people may contract some form of STD by age 25.[10,13] Many of the tragic victims are newborn children, who contract an STD within the uterus or during birth.[13] Of further significance is the large number of asymptomatic carriers and vectors of infection along with the fact that many of the STDs are not required to be reported by law in many states.[1,6,9]

Paul J. Wiesner, M.D., of the United States Public Health Service, has noted:

> Depending upon one's point of view, different terms are utilized to describe the magnitude of the problem of sexually transmitted diseases (STD's) within the United States. Behavioral scientists point out the peculiarities of a society that equips its youth so poorly for sexual development and yet daily encourages them to develop early. Medical sociologists tell how our medical care system has failed to provide accessible and acceptable health services for young people at risk for STD's. Political scientists say that our decision makers and the public

are still unable to respond to an age-old problem rooted in apathy, ignorance, and neglect. Economists decry the waste of health care resources and the loss of productivity from persons with STD's while medical scientists are more impressed with what is not known about the problem than what is known.[14]

Dr. Wiesner (writing in 1980) notes that the incidence of such diseases can be estimated by tabulating data on reportable diseases and then adjusting for underreporting and misdiagnosis and then by cautiously projecting data from special surveys conducted in specific health facilities, and by the utilization of national random surveys of health care encounters. Similarly, the incidence of complications can be estimated by examining random sample surveys of ambulatory care encounters and hospital discharge diagnoses. Some groups have attempted to measure the economic costs of STDs by multiplying the number and length of hospitalizations and the average duration of incapacity by cost figures and productivity factors. However, estimates of economic costs are subject to enormous error as these multipliers themselves are averages of estimates.[14]

Dr. Weisner lists the following statistics within the United States:[14]

- Gonorrhea is still the most reported communicable disease in the United States; reported cases of gonorrhea tripled between 1965 and 1975 — over one million cases were reported in 1979 (with an estimated two million actual cases).
- Sexually transmitted diseases prompt at least five million visits to private physicians' offices each year.
- A study of seven public STD clinics revealed that nongonococcal urethritis is the most common STD in men followed by gonorrhea, pediculosis publis, condyloma acuminata (crabs and warts respectively), and herpes progenitalis in that order.
- For women, the most common STD is gonorrhea followed by trichomoniasis, nonspecific vaginitis, condylomata acuminata (warts), pediculosis publis (crabs), and herpes progenitalis in that order. At least five million women visit STD clinics each year with these conditions. Between 1.6 and 3.2 percent of women visiting family planning clinics have gonorrhea; in outpatient hospital clinics, the figure among women is 3 to 5.6 percent.
- Approximately 1.5 percent of infants have congenital cytomegalovirus infection — of these, 15 percent are left with permanent defects; approximately 3 to 5 percent of neonates have a chlamydial infection, half of whom develop conjunctivitis and 10 to 20 percent of whom develop pneumonia. Approximately three of every 10,000 neonates are infected with herpes simplex virus infections; more than 50 percent of these infants die while half the survivors suffer from chronic morbidity. In 1979, 104 cases of congenital syphilis in infants less than one year of age were reported within the U.S.

The acquired immunodeficiency syndrome (AIDS), which is virtually always fatal, was first diagnosed in 1979 at the UCLA Medical Center. It apparently began in New York City in 1978. By spring 1985 it had been contracted by 9,000 persons in the U.S. and half were already dead; the disease was in 46 states. Two-thirds of the cases were in New York or California — one-half in New York City alone. One year earlier (April 1984) the disease figures in the U.S. were something over 3,000 reported cases and about 1,750 deaths.[15,73,74] The incubation period may range from a few months to perhaps seven or more years. The spread of the disease is frighteningly fast.

Public Knowledge of Sexually Transmitted Diseases

Dr. E.R. Mahoney, professor of sociology at Western Washington University and author of *Human Sexuality* (1983), says that in many respects the Victorian view of sexually transmitted diseases and the ignorance concerning them is still very much present today.[16] To illustrate this, Dr. Mahoney notes, for example, that among college students, overall knowledge of sexually transmitted diseases is quite low, despite the magnitude of the problem and the frequent sexual activity of many young people with a variety of partners.[16] A 1975 study of Michigan teenagers found that 25 percent of the sample believed STDs could be readily contracted from sources other than sexual contact; 14 percent believed that the disappearance of signs and symptoms meant that the disease was "cured" while another quarter of the sample believed that contraction of such a disease provided future immunity against the particular disease contracted.[16] A 1980 study of college students found that only five percent of males and four percent of females noted their parents as their principal source of information on STDs and only 27 percent of the students noted that they had obtained any information on the diseases from their parents.[16]

It is such ignorance and apathy that have largely allowed these diseases to reach epidemic proportions despite cures for almost all of them.[16] Also, negative connotations associated with STDs concerning one's sexual habits and partners and consequent lack of frankness about them help these diseases to continue to spread in alarming proportions.[16]

Doctors James and Stephen McCary, authors of *McCary's Human Sexuality* (1982) state that complete eradication of the sexually transmitted diseases is no longer considered a realistic goal with the present state of technology. Yet, fortunately, scientists continue to expend great efforts in seeking ultimate solutions for the epidemic problem of sexually transmitted diseases within modern society.[17]

1. Acquired Immune Deficiency Syndrome (AIDS)

Acquired immune deficiency syndrome (AIDS) is a virtually 100 percent fatal, sexually transmitted disease caused by the HTLV-3 retrovirus, which most commonly affects homosexual and bisexual males, I.V. drug users, and hemophiliacs receiving contaminated blood. The disease is characterized by profound and persistent fatigue; dyspnea (labored breathing) with minor exertion; low-grade persistent fever; night sweats; unexplained weight loss of more than ten pounds within less than sixty days; generalized lymphadenopathy; dry cough unrelated to smoking or flu; persistent diarrhea and/or bloody stools; ecchymoses, particularly upon limbs; anorexia; opportunistic infections; headaches; a burning sensation upon the posterior tongue; and nausea and/or vomiting.[1-16]

The official surveillance definition for AIDS developed and used by the Centers for Disease Control in Atlanta, Georgia, is as follows:[74]

> The presence of reliably diagnosed disease at least moderately indicative of underlying cellular immunodeficiency (Kaposi's sarcoma) in a patient under 60 years of age, Pneumocystis pneumonia, or other opportunistic infections. Absence of known causes of underlying immunodeficiency and of any other reduced resistance reported to be associated with the disease (immunosuppressive therapy, lymphoreticular malignancy).

Many medical and public health authorities believe that AIDS presently constitutes America's number one health problem. Up to 40 percent of those infected by the virus may develop the disease, there is no vaccine or cure, and the disease is virtually 100 percent fatal after a period of approximately 3 years.[73,84-92]

History

AIDS appears to have been an almost entirely heterosexual disease in central Africa, where it affects men and women in equal numbers.[86,100,101] Epidemiologists believe that the AIDS virus was initially harbored by the African green monkey and then spread to humans.[86,89,100,101] The virus does not appear to affect the monkeys, which may provide a clue for a cure or vaccine; AIDS would not be the first disease to spread from animals to humans (other examples of diseases include jungle yellow fever, rabies, cat-scratch fever, parrot fever, etc.).[1,13,89,100,101]

AIDS was first diagnosed in 1979 at the University of California at Los Angeles Medical Center.[98,100] The first victims were male homosexuals, who presented with pneumocystis carinni pneumonia. The medical profession at that time believed that AIDS was a new disease confined only to homosexuals.[98,100]

Dr. Peter Piot, a Belgian tropical disease expert, has noted that AIDS probably existed within central Africa 20 or more years ago and traveled from Africa to Europe to the Caribbean, then to the United States.[100,101] Dr. James Curran, chief epidemiologist for AIDS research at CDC, notes that AIDS is definitely epidemic within the United States but that gay and bisexual communities are listening to medical authorities and changing their lifestyles by engaging in safe sex, which in essence involves reducing the number of different sexual partners and preventing the exchange of body fluids.[100,101]

Occurrence

At this writing, the Centers for Disease Control in Atlanta, Georgia, and the National Center for Health Statistics have noted an AIDS prevalence of approximately 20,000 reported cases, with a resultant 10,000 deaths, within the United States alone.[102,103] Over 4,000 cases of AIDS have now been reported in at least 40 nations.[104] Every 7 to 9 months, the number of reported AIDS cases within the United States doubles, with 73 percent of patients gay or bisexual males, 17 percent IV drug users, and .7 percent hemophiliacs. Many prostitutes have acquired AIDS and are asymptomatic or symptomatic reservoirs for the disease, infecting many others within a relatively short period of time.[100,101,104] AIDS cases have been reported in 45 states within the United States, and the disease is most common in urban regions with large gay populations such as New York City and San Francisco, where close to 50 percent of the gay population is infected with the HTLV-3 virus, according to some medical and public health authorities.[99,100] It is important to remember that AIDS is not only a disease of the homosexual population; heterosexuals account for approximately 27 percent of cases within the United States to date.[100,101]

The Centers for Disease Control in Atlanta have noted that the *actual* prevalence of AIDS may be 10 times higher than reported to CDC. *The Philadelphia Inquirer* estimated that there may be some 300,000 cases and perhaps 30,000 deaths before a cure and/or vaccine for the disease is found.[102,103,105] It is expected that the number of silent carriers who may infect others may double, from 1 to 2 million to 2 to 4 million, within the next five years unless a vaccine or cure for the disease is found within the near future.[100,101,105]

The Population at Risk

The population at risk for acquired immune deficiency syndrome includes: (1) gay and bisexual males (no instances have been reported among homosexual females) who are sexually promiscuous, with the highest risk in New York City, San Francisco, Los Angeles, and other large cities with large gay and bisexual populations; (2) those sharing contaminated needles and syringes for I.V. recreational drug use*; (3) those using nonparenteral drugs for recreational use, such as marijuana, cocaine, isobutyl nitrate, amyl nitrite, PCP, heroin, and/or ethyl chloride; (4) those with hemophilia-A who received contaminated blood prior to the development of a screening test; (5) offspring of high-risk parents; (6) heterosexual women having regular sexual relations with infected gay or bisexual males; (7) those with a history of recurrent and/or multiple communicable diseases such as gonorrhea, venereal syphilis, viral hepatitis, herpes progenitalis, amebiasis and other forms of enteric infections, as well as those with cytomegalovirus and/or Epstein-Barr viral infections; (8) those with a medical history of chronic malnutrition; (9) those engaged in sexual practices characterized by the ingestion or rectal absorption of feces, urine, seminal fluid, and/or rectal trauma; (10) those using in sexual activity any potentially toxic lubricants that are rapidly absorbed into the circulatory system through the rectal mucosa, such as steroid creams, estrogens, or other chemical preparations such as hand lotions, etc.; (11) some researchers have noted that those with tatoos are at highest risk for AIDS; (12) those sharing toothbrushes, razors, and/or other personal items which may be contaminated with infected blood; and prostitutes, who constitute a special population at risk due to a history of many different sexual partners and the frequency of I.V. and other recreational drug use among them, in addition to a possible history of a variety of acquired sexually transmitted diseases (see number 7, above).[73,84,85,87,89,100,101] Dritz and Goldsmith have noted that both heterosexuals and homosexuals are at risk for AIDS in that oral-genital, procto-genital, and oral-anal sexual practices are not restricted to any single sector of the population or to any specific sexual preference.[70]

A 1986 NBC news special on AIDS noted a study which found that 76 percent of Americans felt that no segment of the population is safe from AIDS.[100] Perhaps 1 to 3 million Americans are infected by the virus.

Of the 40 nations reporting AIDS cases, the largest number of cases exist within the United States, followed by France and Brazil; Haitians are no longer considered a population at risk by the CDC.[99-101,106]

---

*I.V. drug users who acquire AIDS are generally males, in an approximate 4 to 1 ratio to females.

Infectious Etiological Agent

It appears that Dr. Robert Gallo of the National Institutes of Health has discovered the cause of AIDS: the HTLV-3 retrovirus, whose genes are composed of RNA rather than DNA.[15] Dr. Gallo also has the distinction of being the first scientist to discover a human cancer virus; his work has been corroborated by Dr. Luc Montagnier and his associates at the renowned Pasteur Institute of Paris, France.[15] Dr. Gallo found evidence of the HTLV-3 virus in 80 to 90 percent of blood samples from AIDS patients and noted early in his research that a virus was probably the etiological agent of AIDS in that transmission for the disease is similar to that of viral hepatitis-B infections—that is, through urine, feces, and seminal fluid as well as contaminated needles, syringes, blood, and blood products.[15]

Dr. Gallo believes that the ancestor virus of AIDS originated within Africa, since the HTLV-3 virus is endemic in Africa, where it appears to represent the most common cause of human leukemia.[15] Furthermore, Kaposi's sarcoma, a skin cancer to which AIDS patients are prone, has been prevalent in Africa for decades. The prevalence of AIDS within central Africa is as great as it is in New York City and San Francisco.[15]

Dr. Gallo and Dr. Montagnier both noted that the trademark enzyme of retroviruses was frequently present within blood samples of AIDS patients; however, it would be present one week and absent the next.[15] Finally, the explanation was found: The virus was rapidly destroying T-cells within the blood samples, the very cells within which the HTLV-3 virus resided. Once the T-cells within the sample were destroyed, the virus and its enzyme would disappear without a trace. Eventually, Dr. Gallo found a means of keeping AIDS-infected T-cells alive in culture and was then able to identify the virus, which he named HTLV-3 as it was similar to other viruses which he had discovered.[15] Retroviruses are enveloped viruses, formerly best known as agents which can cause malignant neoplasms within various vertebrates; the two previously discovered human retroviruses, human T-cell leukemia virus I and II, are T-cell tropic agents that are associated with acute and chronic T-cell leukemia.[74] The acquired immune deficiency syndrome is a disease in which the underlying abnormality appears to be the depletion of a specific subset of T-cells, those that are OKT4-positive.[74] The definitive method for detecting retrovirus infections is finding a DNA copy of the viral RNA genome integrated into the chromosomal DNA of the infected cell.[74] To date, no vaccine for a retrovirus exists. Creating one will be a major challenge to the scientific community, which hopes to do so within the next few years.[74,77,95,100,101]

Reservoir, Source of Infection, and Mode of Transmission

The reservoir for AIDS is mankind, and it is apparently contracted from the bites of infected green monkeys within central Africa, according to experts at the Harvard University School of Medicine and Public Health.[77,86,100,101]

The source of infection appears to be the viral-laden exudates of infected individuals, communicated during sexual intercourse or by contaminated blood or blood products.[73,74,87,89,100,101] The two fluids considered to be the most highly contagious are blood and seminal fluid; however, the virus has been demonstrated *in all body fluids* — saliva, tears, perspiration, urine, feces, and vaginal secretions.[100,101] Most experts believe that transmission of the virus through tears or saliva from talking, coughing, sneezing, or fomite contamination is highly unlikely; there is no evidence that the disease may be acquired by casual contact.[83,95,104,106] As the AIDS virus is thought to enter the body through broken skin and mucous membranes, such as the oral and/or rectal mucosa, heavy kissing has not been discounted as a potential route of transmission.[95,105] The disease is also spread by contaminated needles and syringes, and may be acquired in utero by babies whose mothers have the disease.[73,74,84,85,87,89,90]

Dr. Harold Jaffe, a CDC epidemiologist, has noted that there is now a 98 percent safety factor for receiving blood or blood products, due to laboratory procedures developed in 1985 to identify contaminated donor blood, which is subsequently discarded.[86,87,89,100,106]

Some scientists believe exposure to the virus is a necessary but perhaps insufficient basis for acquisition of the disease.[107] Thus, acquisition of the disease may require the presence of a co-factor, such as a compromised immune system, a preexisting viral infection (as with cytomegalovirus, Epstein-Barr virus, herpes simplex virus, or hepatitis-B virus), or some other factors.[86,88,107] Other scientists believe that such infections are a result rather than a contributing cause of AIDS infection.[86,88,105] Some investigators believe that the disease may be transmissible through fomites contaminated with blood, such as a shared toothbrush or razor; however, it is known that the disease is not acquired by casual contact, even among family members residing with AIDS patients.[84-106]

To date, there are no reports of family members or medical personnel acquiring the disease through casual contact, as evidenced by clinical experience in medical settings and a study in the *New England Journal of Medicine* (February 1986) of 39 families living with AIDS patients.[84-106]

The University of Pennsylvania School of Medicine has noted that AIDS does *not* appear to be highly contagious, for if it were, there would be many more cases of the disease than presently exist.[83] It must also be noted that one need *not* be promiscuous to get AIDS; one sexual experience with an infected individual must at this time be considered sufficient exposure for potential acquisition of the disease.[100,101,104,105]

Incubation Period

The incubation period for AIDS is idiopathic but is believed to range from several months to perhaps 7 or even 10 years.[83,84,87,89,100,101,104,106]

The typical incubation period is believed to be approximately 3 to 5 years, but it has been documented that patients may present clinically with AIDS just a few months after acquiring the infection.[84,87,89,100-106]

Period of Communicability

The period of communicability for AIDS remains idiopathic, but it is suspected that an infected person may spread the disease whether symptomatic or asymptomatic in a carrier state. Until proven otherwise, the disease must be assumed to be communicable as soon as a patient's blood serum registers positive for the presence of the HTLV-3 virus.[73,83,87,89,88,95-98,100,101]

Susceptibility and Resistance

One's susceptibility to acquired immune deficiency syndrome appears to depend upon viral exposure and infection in conjunction with other cofactors, such as the integrity of one's immune system, nutritional and general health status, use of recreational drugs, level of emotional stress, or history of repeated or multiple sexually transmitted diseases, as already noted in the discussion concerning population at risk. Exactly why some individuals who are infected with the virus or have AIDS-related complex (ARC) develop the disease and others do not is largely unknown.[84,87,89,100,101] What is now known is that those with ARC have perhaps a 40 percent chance of acquiring "full-blown" AIDS, in comparison with previous estimates of 10 percent.[84,87,89,100,101,104,105]

Medical and public health authorities throughout the world state that many individuals have been noted to have generalized lymphadenopathy syndrome (GLS) for a variety of reasons that are not completely understood; yet these individuals do well, clinically speaking.[1,84,100,101]

While individuals with apparently milder cases of the disease and younger patients may fare better than most older patients, the disease is virtually 100 percent fatal within 3 years of diagnosis.[100,101] One patient who was born with AIDS survived for a period of 6 years.[100,101,104,105]

It is known that the HTLV-3 virus can transcend the blood-brain barrier, which makes the development of a vaccine for this disease all the more difficult.[1,84,85,87,89,100,101,105] While HTLV-3 antibodies can transcend the blood-brain barrier, it is difficult to develop effective chemotherapeutic agents that can do the same.[84,85,87,89,100,101]

Signs and Symptoms

There are many diseases that mimic AIDS in their clinical manifestations; however, anyone with one or more of the following signs and symptoms should be carefully examined by his or her family physician, particularly if he or she is among a population at risk for the disease:[73,74,77,84,87,89,100,101,104-107]

- Excessive and persistent fatigue
- Dyspnea with minor exertion for no apparent reason
- A dry cough unrelated to other illness such as a cold, flu, or smoking
- A low-grade and persistent fever
- Persistent night sweats, shaking, and/or chills
- Anorexia, nausea, and/or vomiting
- Unexplained weight loss of 10 or more pounds within 60 days
- Generalized lymphadenopathy syndrome
- Persistent profuse diarrhea and/or bloody stools
- Easily-acquired ecchymoses, particularly upon limbs
- The presence of opportunistic infections, such as Kaposi's sarcoma or pneumocystis carinii pneumonia, cytomegalovirus infections, unusually severe shingles, herpes simplex virus infection, hepatitis virus B infection, thrush, and/or other bacterial infections
- Blurred vision, persistent severe headaches, and/or memory loss
- Persistent unexplained sore throat and/or thrush infection orally
- Unexplained bleeding from any body orifice
- The presence of a positive blood test for AIDS and/or the diagnosis of AIDS in one's sexual partner

Infants acquiring the disease in utero evidence clinical manifestations of the disease shortly after birth (generally to a mother with a medical history of recreational drug abuse, poor diet, high stress, or an otherwise compromised immune system).

Diagnosis

The HTLV-3 Test

The diagnosis of AIDS is based upon the patient's history as a member of a population at risk, clinical manifestations of disease, presence or absence of disease in one's sexual partners, and a positive HTLV-3 blood test indicating infection with this virus.[83,87,89,100,101,105,106] The test is useful in screening the blood of blood donors and may indicate that one may develop AIDS at a later time. However, the test does not constitute a definite diagnosis of AIDS; it merely indicates the presence of antibodies to the HTLV-3 virus, and like many other laboratory tests, may represent a false positive or a false negative.[87,89,100,101,104-106] A negative test does not preclude the possibility for presence and transmission of the virus to others, while a false positive is apt to create considerable anxiety in someone who does not have the disease.[89,100,101,104,106] Furthermore, a positive result has been used by employers, insurance companies, the military, and some governmental agencies in discriminating against individuals with such.[100,101,104-106]

Laboratory Pathophysiology*

The common denominator of AIDS is a profound suppression of cell-mediated immunity, specifically a quantitative and qualitative defect in the T4 inducer or helper subset of T-lymphocytes. Hyperactivity of B-lymphocytes is also characteristic. The clinical manifestations are those of severe and life-threatening opportunistic infections and unusual neoplasms, particularly Kaposi's sarcoma.

1. Profound lymphopenia is one of the most striking features of the immune system of patients with AIDS, with total lymphocyte counts often below 500/mm. This lymphopenia is predominantly due to a loss from the peripheral blood of T-lymphocytes that bear the helper/inducer phenotype defined by the monoclonal antibodies OKT 4 or Leu 3. These subsets can be quantitated through the utilization of fluorescein-conjugated monoclonal antibodies and the utilization of the fluorescence-activated cell sorter. A typical fluorescence-activated cell sorter analysis of a patient with the syndrome shows a marked decrease in the number of cells capable of binding the OKT 4 monoclonal antibody. It is this depletion in the helper/inducer T-lymphocytes that results in a lowering of the helper/suppressor ratio. It is not currently known whether the immunologic dysfunction in this syndrome is due to the imbalance between help and suppression or more directly due to the depletion of T-cell help.[74]

Patients with Kaposi's sarcoma alone have a higher absolute number of T4 lymphocytes than those initially presenting with life-threatening opportunistic infections. This is the immunologic correlate of the observation made in the statistics compiled by the CDC that showed that patients with Kaposi's sarcoma alone have a longer life expectancy than those with opportunistic infections. Thus, those patients who initially present with Kaposi's sarcoma alone may be doing so earlier in the course of a progressive immunodeficiency than those initially presenting with a life-threatening opportunistic infection such as *P. carinii* pneumonia or cryptococcal meningitis.

---

*From the Conference of the Combined Clinical Staffs of the National Institutes of Health at Bethesda, Maryland, on June 23, 1983. Macher, A.M. "Infection in the Acquired Immune Deficiency Syndrome." In Fauci, A.S., moderator, "Acquired Immunodeficiency Syndrome: Epidemiologic, Clinical, Immunologic, and Therapeutic Considerations," *The Annals of Internal Medicine* **100** (January 1984), pp. 92–106.

Although the cause of the basic immunologic lesion remains unknown, the end result, a profound alteration in T-cell function both in vivo and in vitro, is quite evident. In vivo, this alteration in T-cell function may be manifested as the development of neoplasms, the development of opportunistic infections, or the inability to mount a delayed-type hypersensitivity response (cutaneous anergy). Less than 10 percent of patients have shown the ability to develop a positive skin test when tested with appropriate recall antigens. This inability reflects a profound degree of cellular immune dysfunction. However, as Siegal has noted, this function may be variably intact in early stages of the syndrome.[74]

Virtually all in-vitro measurements of T-lymphocyte function are decreased in patients with the syndrome. These measurements include the responses to nonspecific signals delivered by mitogens as well as responses to the specific signals delivered by soluble antigens such as tetanus toxoid or alloantigens expressed upon the surface of allogeneic lymphocytes (mixed lymphocyte reaction).[74]

The T-lymphocyte competence can also be assessed in vitro by the measurement of certain percent-cell effector functions such as providing help to B-lymphocytes or eliciting a virus-specific cytotoxic lymphocyte response. In both of these variables, patients have been shown to be markedly deficient. When assayed in a system for measuring immunoglobulin production in which normal helper/inducer cells were present, the suppressor/cytotoxic subpopulation of lymphocytes from the patients appeared to function normally. Similarly, cytotoxic lymphocyte function could be restored to normal simply by the addition of interleukin-2 to culture. Phenotypically, however, these cytotoxic/suppressor lymphocytes have been shown to be activated in vivo because they express certain surface antigens associated with an activated stage of the cell cycle. Whether this in-vivo activation of suppressor/cytotoxic T-lymphocytes is related to the immunopathogenesis of the syndrome or is simply part of the normal in-vivo response to viral infection remains to be determined.[74]

The peripheral blood B-lymphocytes of patients with the syndrome are characterized by an enormous degree of polyclonal activation. This activation is shown serologically as elevated levels of total immunoglobulin, predominantly IgG and IgA. In addition, immune complexes have been shown in the sera of most patients with the syndrome. Finally, there is an increased number of peripheral blood B-cells that spontaneously secrete immunoglobulin reflecting a polyclonal activation. The B-cells in such an activated state are refractory to subsequent primary activation signals. These findings are most likely due to the activation and transformation of peripheral blood B-lymphocytes by an agent such as Epstein-Barr virus in the absence of the normal regulatory T-lymphocyte influences.

Paradoxically, this polyclonal B-cell activation is accompanied by an inability to mount a de novo serologic response to the primary protein antigen keyhole limpet hemocyanin. This fact has important clinical implications regarding the ability of patients either to develop specific humoral immunity or to use the development of such immunity as a clinical test for infection (serologic diagnosis). Serologic responses to recall antigens appear to be highly variable.[74]

2. Other markers of immune dysfunction. — In addition to these abnormalities of T- and B-cell function, patients have other serologic markers of altered immune function. These markers include the presence of a heat-labile form of alpha interferon, elevated alpha-1 thymosin levels, and the presence of substances capable of suppressing the in-vitro immune responses of normal lymphocytes.[74]

3. Host responses to viral infections. (From Dr. Alain H. Rook, Research Investigator, Division of Virology, National Center for Drugs and Biologics, Food and Drug Administration.) Cytomegalovirus and Epstein-Barr virus infections may simulate the clinical and immunologic abnormalities seen in this syndrome. For example, lymphadenopathy and prolonged fever are common during their cytomegalovirus or Epstein-Barr virus infections, and depressed responsiveness to certain T-cell mitogens occurs during cytomegalovirus infection. Also, transplant patients with cytomegalovirus infection have an enhanced susceptibility to other opportunistic infections.[74]

In the study discussed by Dr. Rook, at initial presentation, patients with AIDS, chronic lymphadenopathy syndrome, and asymptomatic cohorts had throat, urine, blood, and any suspicious skin or mucous membrane lesions cultured for cytomegalovirus, Epstein-Barr virus, herpes simplex virus, and varicella-zoster virus. In addition, virus-specific antibody determinations were done, including anticytomegalovirus IgM and IgG and anti–Epstein-Barr virus capsid antigen, early antigen, and nuclear antigen.[74]

Cytomegalovirus was isolated from one or more sites from nearly all patients with AIDS or chronic lymphadenopathy, but cytomegalovirus viremia was found only in the group with the former. Anticytomegalovirus IgM, indicative of recently onset cytomegalovirus infection, was found in 15 of 16 serum samples from patients with AIDS, 4 of 7 samples from those with lymphadenopathy, and none of 5 samples from asymptomatic homosexual men. Combining the results of culture and IgM serologic findings, all patients with AIDS or chronic lymphadenopathy had evidence of active or recent onset of cytomegalovirus infection.[74]

Epstein-Barr virus infection was nearly universal in these same patients. Twenty-five of twenty-seven patients had Epstein-Barr virus isolated from throat washings. Antibody to Epstein-Barr virus early antigens, detectable only during primary or reactivation infection, was found in the sera of 50 percent of these patients, including one of the two patients who were culture-negative, thus providing culture or serologic evidence of active Epstein-Barr virus infection in 96 percent of patients with AIDS. The Epstein-Barr virus infections must have resulted from reactivation of latent virus, because all of these patients had antibodies to Epstein-Barr virus nuclear antigen.[74]

Herpes simplex and varicella-zoster virus infection, in contrast, were much less common, being documented in 6 of 28 and 1 of 28 patients, respectively. With regard to the relative frequency of herpes virus infections, AIDS patients do not resemble other populations with depressed-mediated immunity. For instance, among bone marrow transplant recipients who have a high frequency of all herpes virus infections, herpes simplex virus and varicella-zoster virus are more frequent, whereas cytomegalovirus and Epstein-Barr virus are significantly less frequent than in the AIDS patients in this study. These findings imply that immunosuppression alone is unlikely to account for the prevalence of cytomegalovirus and Epstein-Barr virus infections in AIDS.[74]

The integrity of specific and nonspecific antiviral cellular immune responses was studied, in view of the universal occurrence of cytomegalovirus infection in patients with AIDS. In bone marrow and renal transplant patients, HLA-restricted cytotoxic T-cells and natural killer cells are the cells whose immune functions correlate most significantly with recovery from cytomegalovirus infections. During acute cytomegalovirus infections, there is usually an increase in this cytotoxicity mediated by both enhanced natural killer cell activity and cytotoxic T-cells, the latter cell type being found in the circulation only during acute infection.[74]

In light of these observations, it is noteworthy that all of the patients with AIDS whom Dr. Rook studied had absent cytomegalovirus-specific cytotoxic T-cell activity in the presence of active infection with cytomegalovirus, and most had depressed natural killer cell activity as well. This deficiency in cytotoxic T-cell activity may underlie the heightened susceptibility of persons with AIDS, not only to cytomegalovirus, but also to other opportunistic infectious agents.[74]

To understand the basis for the deficient cytotoxic T-cell activity, the capacity of lymphocytes of patients was examined with respect to their capacity to produce and to respond to various immunoregulatory lymphokines that are important for the normal differentiation and maturation of cytotoxic T-cells. Phytohemagglutinin stimulation of these lymphocytes resulted in markedly reduced release of interleukin-2 and gamma interferon compared to the levels produced by the lymphocytes from healthy heterosexual subjects.

In addition, although the natural killer cell activity of normal lymphocytes utilizing K562 cells as targets was consistently augmented by beta interferon or alpha interferon, as is commonly seen, lymphocytes of AIDS patients were refractory to this immune-enhancing effect of the interferons. In contrast to the lack of effect of beta or alpha interferon, cultivation of these lymphocytes in vitro with highly purified interleukin-2 resulted in a marked augmentation of both natural killer cell and cytomegalovirus-specific cytotoxic activities and was associated with a restored ability to release gamma interferon. Although the mechanism through which interleukin-2 enhances these important antiviral immune responses is uncertain, it may include the effect of interleukin-2 on gamma interferon release because gamma interferon is known to be required for cytotoxic T-cell differentiation.[74]

At the present time, it is clear that patients with AIDS have clinical effects due to a profound defect in T-cell immunity. The present data suggest that if an exogenous source of interleukin-2 were provided, abnormalities in important cell-mediated antiviral immune responses would be corrected. Potentially, this action could lead to recovery from the many devastating opportunistic infections which commonly afflict these patients.[74]

Disease Patterns of AIDS Patients

Clearly, the commonest manifestation of the syndrome, comprising 51 percent of the 2,008 patients reported to the CDC within the United States by August, 1983, was *P. carinii* pneumonia without Kaposi's sarcoma. Kaposi's sarcoma without *P. carinii* pneumonia formed the next largest group, accounting for 27 percent of patients, while 7 percent of patients had both Kaposi's sarcoma and *P. carinii* pneumonia. Sixteen percent of patients had other opportunistic infections without *P. carinii* pneumonia or Kaposi's sarcoma.[74]

1. **Chronic lymphadenopathy syndrome.** — The CDC has defined the chronic unexplained lymphadenopathy syndrome in homosexual men as: Lymphadenopathy of at least three months' duration involving two or more extrainguinal sites and confirmed upon physical examination; absence of any current illness or drug utilization known to cause lymphadenopathy; and the presence of reactive hyperplasia within a lymph node, if a biopsy is performed. The relationship of this syndrome to AIDS is presently unclear.[74]

2. **Oral candidiasis** is commonly seen, and extension of lesions distally leads to esophageal erosions; patients have dysphagia, odynophagia, and retrosternal burning. Barium studies (esophagrams) show mucosal ulcerations, and samples from esophageal biopsies show invasive candidiasis.[74]

3. **Herpes virus infections** are common in AIDS patients; both primary and recurrent herpes simplex virus infections may appear as vesicular lesions upon erythema based within the oral, genital, or perineal

regions. Recurrences often involve extensive genital and perirectal ulcerations but may also involve the esophageal and tracheobronchial mucosa.[74]

4. **Cytomegalovirus infections** have been isolated from several patient sites, including throat washings, urine, and blood from nearly all patients studied at the National Institutes of Health (NIH) Clinical Center. Fevers, granulocytopenia, lymphocytopenia, thrombocytopenic purpura, maculopapular rashes, interstitial pneumonia, chorioretinitis, encephalitis, and ulcerative gastrointestinal lesions are all potential manifestations of cytomegalovirus (CMV) infections in patients with AIDS.[74]

5. **Epstein-Barr Virus** has been isolated from the throat washings and peripheral blood lymphocytes of virtually all patients. Although the clinical significance of this finding is still unclear, it may relate to the tendency of these patients to develop lymphoid malignancies.[74]

6. **Mycobacterium Avium-Intercellulare** is a ubiquitous environmental saprophyte that, in the past, had rarely been shown to be a cause of disseminated disease. However, *M. avium*-intracellulare has been a common pathogen in patients with AIDS, suggesting that these patients have an unusual immunologic lesion that selectively predisposes them to this heretofore rare mycobacterial pathogen. *Mycobacterium avium*-intracellulare is typically shown in and cultured from bone marrow, lymph node, and liver biopsy samples from patients with AIDS. More strikingly, blood cultures from 8 patients at the NIH Clinical Center have grown *M. avium*-intracellulare and these patients are, therefore, mycobactermic. Histopathologic findings from biopsy samples commonly show a histiocytic process as true granulomata are often poorly formed or absent. Acid-fast stains show large clusters of mycobacteria within the cytoplasm of the histiocytes. These clusters, or "globi," of acid-fast mycobacteria are reminiscent of those seen in patients with lepromatous leprosy.[74]

7. **Diffuse pneumonitis** is a common manifestation of AIDS and may be caused by cytomegalovirus, *Cryptococcus neoformans, M. avium*-intracellulare, and even Kaposi's sarcoma when intra-alveolar hemorrhage is associated with pulmonary Kaposi's sarcoma. However, the commonest cause of diffuse pneumonitis is *P. carinii*.[74]

8. **Pneumocystis carinii pneumonia**, in patients with AIDS, differs from the disease seen in other groups of immunosuppressed patients. In AIDS patients, *Pneumocystis carinii* pneumonia is characterized by a subacute and insidious onset; the patient usually complains of a mild cough or chest discomfort of 2 to 10 weeks duration. Chest radiographs show subtle infiltrates, and often the patient has minimal hypoxemia with arterial blood gases in the range of 80 to 95mm Hg on room air.

Histopathologic findings show pneumocyst organisms in large numbers, and not uncommonly, large numbers are found within the bronchial lavages of patients. Furthermore, *P. carinii* pneumonia often presents within the setting of other opportunistic infections occurring at the same time. Thus, in addition to bacterial, mycobacterial, fungal, and viral cultures, rapid special stains have been utilized including toluidine blue O, Gram Weigert, or methanamine silver.[74]

9. **Central nervous system disease** affects many AIDS patients and may present as a progressive idiopathic encephalopathy, relapsing cryptococcal meningitis, mass lesions due to *Toxoplasma gondii*, progressive multifocal leukoencephalopathy, and central nervous system lymphoma. The idiopathic encephalopathy is characterized by a slowly progressive dementia which often becomes incapacitating. Computed tomographic examination of the brain often shows no focal lesions, but the lateral ventricles may be enlarged. Results of brain biopsy or autopsy show nonspecific inflammation, often with demyelinization, but no etiologic agent. In patients with progressive multifocal leukoencephalopathy, computed tomography may show intra-axial hypodense focal lesions, and tissue from brain biopsy sample will show characteristic inclusion cells utilizing the immunohistochemical staining technique.[74]

10. **Cryptococcal meningitis** is a relatively common complication in AIDS patients; however, cryptococcal meningitis is often part of a disseminated process with positive blood and bone marrow cultures. The disease often recurs despite apparently adequate therapy.[74]

11. **Toxoplasma gondii and lymphoma** represent the commonest causes of mass lesions within the central nervous system of AIDS patients. Patients with toxoplasma infection develop fever and focal neurologic signs. Computed tomographic examination with contrast typically reveals single or multiple enhancing intra-axial mass lesions. Unfortunately, serologic findings have not been useful diagnostically, utilizing the Sabin Feldman dye test of IgM-enzyme-linked immunosorbent assay titers. Therefore, definitive diagnosis requires showing the tachyzoite in tissue sections or by isolating the organism through intraperitoneal mouse injections from a tissue that does not ordinarily contain the dormant cyst.[74]

12. **Chorioretinitis** is a common complication in AIDS patients. Although occasionally patients will present with *T. gondii* retinitis (diagnosed by vitrectomy), the commonest cause of progressive chorioretinitis is cytomegalovirus. Initially, the lesions are asymptomatic as perivascular exudates and hemorrhages are seen. However, as the lesions enlarge and begin to involve macula, vision becomes compromised. At autopsy, numerous cytomegalovirus inclusion cells are shown in the necrotic retinal, choroidal, and optic nerve tissues.[74]

13. Persistent or Recurrent Diarrhea is a frequent problem among AIDS patients, who may have several loose stools per day; others may have copious volumes of watery diarrhea that can reach 15 liters per day. Homosexuals with AIDS may have a range of bowel problems due to the enteric organisms that cause symptomatic disease within the homosexual population in general, including *Entameoba histolytica* and *Giardia lamblia*, as well as species of Shigella, Salmonella, and Campylobacter. Appropriate antimicrobial treatment that eliminates these pathogens often fails to eliminate the copious watery diarrhea. Some patients with persistent watery stools have cryptosporidiosis. *Cryptosporidium* is an enteric coccidia that attaches to the epithelial surface of the small and large intestine; it ordinarily infects animals but occasionally causes a self-limiting diarrheal illness in immunocompetent humans. The oocyst form of the protozoan is found in stool specimens utilizing a sucrose flotation method. Although thorough evaluation has in some patients shown celiac disease, cytomegalovirus lesions, *M. avium*-intracellulare infiltration of the bowel wall, or gastrointestinal Kaposi's sarcoma, many patients with persistent diarrhea have no demonstrable pathogen despite careful stool examination, endoscopic examination, small bowel biopsy, and autopsy.[74]*

14. Kaposi's sarcoma and miscellaneous neoplasms.** — Two types of malignancy have been seen with increased frequency in patients with AIDS: Kaposi's sarcoma and malignant lymphomas of several histologic types, including Burkitt's lymphoma, immunoblastic lymphoma (a subtype of Rappaport's diffuse histiocytic lymphoma), lymphoblastic lymphoma, and Hodgkin's disease. These lymphomas are histologic subtypes with diverse cells of origin, including B-cells, T-cells, and dendritic cells (monocyte-macrophage). Rarely do patients have both Kaposi's sarcoma and malignant lymphoma. Furthermore, the incidence of two other malignancies has increased in one of the groups which are at high risk of developing AIDS, namely, male homosexuals. These malignancies are squamous cell carcinoma of the tongue and cloacogenic carcinoma of the rectum. The latter arises in the transitional epithelium at the anorectal junction and accounts for 3 percent of all rectal cancer; it has the same epidemiology as rectal cancer of other histologic types. The occurrence of these two malignancies in young homosexual men was recognized in the early 1970s prior to the appearance of AIDS within the gay community. Therefore, it is felt that tongue and rectal cancers are not related to the

---

*This study was conducted upon 2,008 AIDS patients reported to the CDC within the United States by August, 1983, prior to the discovery of the HTLV-3 virus which apparently causes AIDS in April, 1984, by Dr. Robert Gallo of the National Institutes of Health in Bethesda, Maryland.

**From Dr. Dan L. Longo, head of the Experimental Immunology Section, Medical Branch, National Cancer Institute.

acquired immune deficiency syndrome but coincidentally occur in a common risk group.[74]

The magnitude of the problem of Kaposi's sarcoma is revealed within the following statistics:[74] Approximately 34 percent of AIDS patients have developed Kaposi's sarcoma and nearly 28 percent of these patients have died. When the incidence of lymphoma in these patients (3 percent to 4 percent) is added to that of Kaposi's sarcoma, nearly 40 percent of the patients have developed a malignancy.[74] This number is over twice the incidence of malignancy in patients with other primary and secondary immunodeficiency states.[74]

The four clinical subtypes are classified upon the degree of local invasiveness and organ or node involvement. *Nodular Kaposi's sarcoma* consists of blue or brown nodules or plaques confined to the skin (generally starting upon the legs; however, lesions may be numerous and widespread). Autotransplantation has been demonstrated along with Koebner's phenomenon (spread of the lesions to sites of trauma). *Florid and infiltrative Kaposi's sarcoma* subtypes are locally destructive lesions, with the former generally causing fungating skin lesions and the latter deep tissue and bone invasion by direct extension from the skin. *Disseminated or lymphadenopathic Kaposi's sarcoma* subtype is defined as any distant spread to visceral organs and/or lymph nodes.[74]

There are two essential features of the histopathologic mechanism of Kaposi's sarcoma regardless of the clinical syndrome: vascular proliferation (vascular spaces need not be lined by endothelium), and spindle-shaped neoplastic cells in a network of reticulin fibers that appear to be of endothelial origin by virtue of their binding of antibody to factor VIII and proliferating in vitro in response to endothelial growth factor. Tumors may be subcategorized based upon the atypia of the cells and the abundance of vascular formations. Skin involvement tends to be intradermal and lesions occurring within other epithelial-lined organs tend to be within the submucosa.[74]

Epidemiology: In addition to patients with AIDS, Kaposi's sarcoma is seen in elderly Jewish and Italian men (incidence .03 cases per 100,000 people), African children or young adults within the same regions where Burkitt's lymphoma is prevalent, and among transplant recipients. These nonepidemic forms of Kaposi's sarcoma have a 10 percent incidence of extracutaneous organ involvement, in comparison to a 72 percent incidence of extracutaneous organ involvement for the epidemic form of Kaposi's sarcoma. That 72 percent includes lymph nodes, gastrointestinal tract, and lungs. Although relatively uncommon, the latter can result in severe physiologic compromise. All segments of the gastrointestinal tract, from mouth to anus, may be involved, and there is a correlation between the presence of oropharyngeal lesions and other gastrointestinal sites of the disease. Approximately 5 percent of the patients with Kaposi's sarcoma have extracutaneous organ system disease in the absence of skin involvement.[74]

The median survival of patients with nonepidemic Kaposi's sarcoma is approximately 13 years (range of 2 months to 50 years), with the common causes of death being cardiac failure, secondary malignancies, sepsis from infected skin lesions, and hemorrhaging. Approximately one-third of patients (up to 37 percent) develop a secondary neoplasm.[74]

The etiology is idiopathic. The disappearance of the disease in patients where the immunodeficiency can be reversed links the cause to immune depression and supports the proposition that the disease may be reactive rather than a malignant transformation. Abundant data link cytomegalovirus to the nonepidemic forms of this disease. The high frequency of the HLA-DR-5 allele in one series of Kaposi's sarcoma related to AIDS (63 percent of patients versus 23 percent in the normal male homosexual population) implies that immune response gene phenomena may contribute to the development of this disease. The analysis of Kaposi's sarcoma cell lines may clarify the pathogenesis of this complication of AIDS.[74]

15. Abnormalities in Immune Function include *lymphopenia,* predominately due to a selective defect in the helper/inducer subset (OKT-4, Leu 3) of T-lymphocytes; *decreased in-vivo T-cell function* — susceptibility to neoplasms, opportunistic infections, and decreased delayed-type hypersensitivity; *altered in-vitro T-cell function* — decreased blast transformation, alloreactivity, specific and nonspecific cytotoxicity along with decreased ability to provide help to B-lymphocytes; *polyclonal B-cell activation* — elevated levels of total serum immunoglobulins and circulating immune complexes; inability to mount a de novo serologic response antigen; increased numbers of spontaneous immunoglobulin-secreting cells; and refractoriness to normal in-vitro signals for B-cell activation.[74]

Treatment

Unfortunately, at this time, there is no cure or vaccine for AIDS. Good personal hygiene, an excellent diet, sufficient sleep and rest, and prevention and treatment of opportunistic infections, the management of diarrhea, and efforts to improve immune system functioning, along with halting the action of the AIDS virus, constitute present treatment efforts in large measure.[87,89,5,100,101,104,106]

A number of treatment methods have been employed using radiation, surgery, and chemotherapy with such agents as HPA-23, Ribavirin, Interleukin-2, Azidothymidine, Cyclosporin A, Interferon, and Compound S in an attempt to reduce the activity of the AIDS virus and bolster the patient's immune system functioning. While some of these agents show promise, there is no drug or other form of treatment currently known that cures the disease or completely restores immune system functioning. Some experts believe that AIDS patients may have to be maintained on viral-suppressant chemotherapeutic agents for the rest of their lives.[87,89,100,101,104,106]

Below we will discuss treatment of AIDS and related infections as reported during the Conference of the Combined Clinical Staffs of the National Institutes of Health, June 23, 1983.*

Because AIDS patients die primarily due to opportunistic infection, prognosis could presumably be improved either by developing more effective antimicrobial treatment or by reconstituting the defective immune response. Given the broad range of life-threatening infections to which these patients are susceptible, the latter approach has more theoretical appeal. Unfortunately, to date no patient has successfully regained immunocompetence either spontaneously or due to a therapeutic manipulation. Thus, treatment must be directed at controlling infections and neoplasms until a means for achieving immunologic reconstitution can be developed.

Treatment for some opportunistic infections, such as *P. carinii* pneumonia, cryptococcal meningitis, candida esophagitis, and mucocutaneous herpes simplex disease, is often effective in these patients. These infections can be fatal, however, and even when effectively treated, they tend to recur. In contrast, several of the frequently occurring infections are untreatable with currently available regimens. These include disseminated *M. avium*-intracellulare, disseminated cytomegalovirus, and cryptosporidiosis.[74]

1. Pneumocystic infections. — A comparison of *P. carinii* pneumonia in patients with and without the syndrome between 1979 and 1983 has shown that mortality in these two patient groups is almost identical at 30 percent. If the rapidity of response to drug therapy is compared in the two patient groups, there is no major difference in the number of days required for the patients to defervesce or for the chest radiograph to begin to clear. However, patients with AIDS are much less effective in completely resolving their infection and often manifest cough, shortness of breath, substantial hypoxemia, and disease relapse after 10 to 14 days of pentamidine or trimethoprim-sulfamethoxazole treatment, which is rarely the case in patients with malignant neoplasms and *P. carinii* pneumonia. Biopsy specimens from many of these patients after 14 to 28 days of treatment often yield results that do not differ substantially from the initial biopsy specimen in terms of cellular infiltrate, alveolar exudate, or quantity of organisms. Whether a longer course of treatment or combined drug therapy would decrease the frequency of persistent symptoms or disease relapses is not known.[74]

*From Macher, A.M. "Infection in the Acquired Immune Deficiency Syndrome." In Fanci, A.S., moderator, "Acquired Immunodeficiency Syndrome: Epidemiological, Clinical, Immunologic, and Therapeutic Considerations," *The Annals of Internal Medicine* **100** (January 1984).

A striking feature of drug therapy for pneumocystosis in AIDS has been the extraordinarily high frequency of adverse reactions to trimethoprim-sulfamethoxazole. When therapeutic doses of this drug are utilized, hypersensitivity rashes develop in 30 percent of patients, and leukopenia (including a decline of greater than 3,000 leukocytes/mm) develops in 30 percent compared to less than 5 percent for each complication in patients without the syndrome. Adverse reactions appear to be unusually frequent when prophylactic doses are utilized as well, limiting this drug's potential for preventing this major infectious complication.[74]

2. Oropharyngeal candidiasis and candida esophagitis in patients with AIDS have been relatively amenable to conventional antifungal treatment. Oral candida may resolve when nystatin liquid or clotrimazole troches are utilized every 4 hours. Often, however, oral ketoconazole or intravenous amphotericin B are needed to resolve the lesions. Oral candidiasis usually recurs as soon as treatment is stopped; therefore, patients need to be maintained on oral ketoconazole or nystatin for the duration of their lifetime. *Candida esophagitis* responds to either oral ketoconazole or intravenous amphotericin B quite promptly. Symptoms resolve within several days, and after 14 days, endoscopic examination usually shows complete resolution of lesions. Relapses appear to be particularly common after ketoconazole therapy.[74]

3. Mucocutaneous herpes simplex virus infections usually respond promptly to a 7 to 10 day course of intravenous acyclovir. Viral shedding ceases within several days and lesions epithelialize. Recurrences in the same area are very common in patients with AIDS.[74]

4. Cryptococcal disease is difficult to treat in AIDS patients. Many are leukopenic and cannot tolerate flucytosine therapy without developing even more serious decreases in leukocyte production. Treatment with amphotericin B (0.6 mg/kg body weight or 0.3 mg/kg body weight) for long courses up to a total dose of 2 to 3 g is usually associated with a symptomatic response, sterilization of blood and spinal fluid, and reduction in cryptococcal antigen titers. However, after amphotericin B is stopped, relapses are quite common, and at autopsy, active cryptococcal disease can usually be found despite apparently adequate treatment.[74]

5. Cryptosporidiosis has been treated with over 30 different drugs, including metronidazole, quinacrine, trimethoprim-sulfamethoxazole, and tetracycline. None of these compounds has succeeded in decreasing the volume of diarrhea or the quantity of cryptosporidia being passed. Symptomatic relief can be obtained in some patients by utilizing tincture of opium, diphenoxylate, or perhaps cholestyramine. In many patients with cryptosporidiosis, the diarrhea does *not* abate despite aggressive symptomatic therapy.[74]

6. Disseminated cytomegalovirus disease has not responded to intravenous acyclovir or vidarabine. The quanity of circulating virus is not substantially diminished, and organ dysfunction, such as chorioretinitis, is not ameliorated.[74]

7. Toxoplasmosis. — Sulfadiazine and pyrimethamine have appeared to be effective in limiting the progression of toxoplasmosis in some, but not all, patients with AIDS. Because these drugs suppress bone marrow, they are administered with great difficulty to many patients with the syndrome who are leukopenic to begin with. For patients who do respond, antitoxoplasma therapy probably needs to be continued for life.

8. Nonepidemic forms of Kaposi's sarcoma have generally been treated with localized radiotherapy with x-rays, or more extended field or total body electron beam radiotherapy because most patients have localized disease. This treatment achieves a complete response in 93 percent to 100 percent of patients. Those patients with more aggressive or advanced diesease have shown high response rates to a wide range of chemotherapeutic agents utilized singly and in combination; however, the rarity of the tumor has meant that most treatment reports involve a small number of patients. The median survival of patients with nonepidemic Kaposi's sarcoma is 13 years (range of 2 months to 50 years), and the common causes of death are cardiac failure, secondary malignancies, sepsis from infected skin lesions, and/or hemorrhaging, with up to 37 percent of patients developing secondary tumors.[74]

9. The epidemic form, associated with AIDS, has not been as successfully treated as the nonepidemic form of Kaposi's sarcoma. Over 60 patients have received some type of interferon. Approximately 10 percent of the patients have had complete responses, and another 20 percent have had short-duration partial responses. Two small series of patients treated with chemotherapy have been reported utilizing single agents and combinations. The studies have not been randomized, and in general, patients with more aggressive disease have been given the combinations. Responses are common, but 30 percent of all reported patients have died, and the projected 2-year survival is only 30 percent. There have been no long-term, disease-free survivors (longest remission, 12 months). The causes of death in most patients have been overwhelming opportunistic infections and irreversible cachexia and wasting. Tumor-related deaths comprise only about 25 percent of the total.

The cause of Kaposi's sarcoma is idiopathic; the disappearance of the disease within patients where the immunodeficiency can be reversed links the cause to immune depression and supports the proposition that the disease may be reactive rather than a malignant transformation.[74] Abundant data link cytomegalovirus to the nonepidemic forms of the disease.[74]

The ultimate success in controlling the malignancies associated with AIDS most likely depends upon the reversal of the immune dysfunction.[74]

10. Investigative means to reconstitute immunologic competence. — Because antimicrobial treatment is often ineffective in patients with AIDS, a major thrust of current investigations is to find effective means to reconstitute immunologic competence. If a virus or other infectious agent attacks cells which are immunologically competent, such as lymphocytes, one possible intervention would be to treat the patient with an antiviral drug or an interferon product to abolish the causative agent, if the immune defect was caused by the persistence of this agent. To date, a few patients have been treated with prolonged courses of acyclovir or vidarabine, but improved immunologic response has not resulted. Interferon products have been utilized to prevent viral infection of leukocytes and thus to potentially restore immunocompetence. The trials of alpha interferon have not yet been uniformly successful in restoring immune function, though some trials have shown modest antitumor effect.[74]

As noted previously, the lymphocytes from AIDS patients are deficient in their ability to produce gamma interferon or interleukin-2. Gamma interferon has the ability to enhance cytotoxic lymphocyte function. Interleukin-2 has a role in the proliferation and differentiation of T-lymphocytes, and it also stimulates gamma interferon production. Therapeutic trials with these compounds are currently underway in our attempts to restore immunocompetence.

If rejection phenomena could be overcome, it would seem more fruitful to provide patients with immunocompetent cells which could populate the appropriate sites and exert the proper biological effects on immune response, thus obviating the need to identify and quantitate all of their humoral products. An unusual opportunity to assess transplantation was provided by a patient at the NIH who had a healthy identical twin. The transfer of 3×10^{10} mature lymphocytes to the patient without previous immunologic ablation resulted in a modest increase in several immunologic parameters, including skin test hypersensitivity and absolute OKT 4+ lymphocyte count. However, this increase was transient. Subsequent transfer of 3×10^{10} bone marrow cells with periodic transfers of mature peripheral lymphocytes resulted in a more sustained increase in skin test hypersensitivity and OKT 4+ T lymphocytes, but these increases were also only temporary, and the patient subsequently developed Kaposi's sarcoma, progressive cytomegalovirus chorioretinitis, and repeated bouts of *P. carinii* pneumonia, which led ultimately to his death, proving that from a clinical standpoint, he had *not* been immunologically reconstituted. Clearly, this patient had persistent infections or immunologic abnormalities that prevented normal cells from restoring immunocompetence.[74]

AIDS Vaccine Research

Regrettably, major pharmaceutical firms within the United States have given AIDS research a low priority; an exception has been Hoffman-

LaRoche Corporation, which is more active in this regard and has developed an excellent educational program for television featuring the nation's leading AIDS experts ("AIDS — Profile of An Epidemic").[100] According to L. Patrick Gage, vice-president for exploratory research at Hoffman-LaRoche, "Right now there is limited commercial opportunity. The reason we are involved is that there is a medical need to be involved."[100,106]

Dr. Jeffrey Lawrence of the Cornell University Medical Center notes that an AIDS vaccine is probably 2 or more years away, in that only recently has a vaccine been developed for a retrovirus.[100,101] Professor Natan Trainin of the Weizman Institute of Science has noted that the thymus hormones of calves appear to improve the immune system of AIDS patients and slow the progress of the disease.[105] The small green African monkeys who perhaps created the disease may hold the key to a vaccine, since the monkeys themselves fare well with the disease.[86,87,89,100,101,105]

The Social Effects of AIDS

Initially, AIDS was called the "Gay Plague," and some AIDS patients were refused care and treatment by physicians, nurses, police, ambulance personnel, laboratory technicians, and other medical personnel.[73,87,89,100,101] The general public became concerned about giving blood, and as a result, the national blood supply fell to a very low level.[100,101] Hemophiliacs were concerned about accepting blood (which constitutes an important part of their treatment, since hemophiliacs are more likely to die from hemorrhaging than from any other single cause of mortality, at least in their younger years.[100,101]

Many gay people with AIDS were disowned by their families, fired from their jobs, denied subsequent employment opportunities, denied medical care, or abandoned by their friends. They reacted to the diagnosis with shock, disbelief, depression, anger, anxiety, guilt, loss of self-respect, fear, and a concern for not only their health but their very lives.[73,87,89,100,101] The patients of AIDS tended to react as one might have reacted to a diagnosis of cancer perhaps 10 or more years ago.[100] The armed forces at one point discussed a plan to treat and retain heterosexuals but to dismiss homosexuals without treating them because they could "bankrupt the military."

Questions of confidentiality and the legal rights of AIDS patients presently constitute very important ethical issues in society. Oncologists used to treating dying cancer patients, who are often elderly, find it upsetting to see AIDS death among individuals within the prime of life.[100,101]

The gay community has noted that only when it became apparent that the disease was affecting heterosexuals as well did the public become concerned to a considerable degree, and that the government did much too little too late in its effort to solve this problem, due to the traditionally unpopular lifestyle of most of its victims.[73,87,89,100,101]

Due to the recognition that AIDS is primarily a "gay or bisexual disease," at least in the United States, many gay and bisexual men have reduced their number of sexual partners and are cooperating with public health authorities in efforts to prevent the disease and to raise money to find a cure or a vaccine for the disease at the earliest possible date.[73,87,89,100]

AIDS has become, in the opinion of many, America's number one health problem; given its rapidly increasing prevalence and its extremely high death rate, it is easy to see why public health professionals and all concerned citizens are anxiously awaiting a cure and/or vaccine for the disease.[73,95,100,101,106] In view of the frequent updates in AIDS treatment and statistics, it is important that the public remain alert to current and reliable media information.

2. Chancroid

Also known as *soft chancre* or *ulcus molle*, chancroid is an acute localized autoinoculable sexually transmitted disease caused by the streptobacillus of Ducrey and characterized by necrotizing ulcerations at the inoculation site, lymphadenopathy, and suppuration of the regional lymph nodes.[10,33]

Occurrence

There are no particular differences in the incidence of chancroid according to age, race, or sex except as determined by sexual habits.[6] Chancroid is geographically widespread and relatively common in seaports and urban areas; the incidence is sometimes higher than that of venereal syphilis in military forces and tropical regions.[6,8] The actual number of cases of chancroid occurring every year cannot be accurately determined, as a definitive diagnosis of this condition is often not attempted; a diagnosis of chancroid is frequently applied to genital lesions which improve with sulfonamide chemotherapy and in which *Treponema pallidum* cannot be demonstrated.[33,46] The disease is encountered in the West Indies, North Africa, and the Orient, particularly among populations of lower socioeconomic status; it is also prevalent in the eastern part of the United States. Some medical authorities claim that is more frequent in blacks than whites; other disagree.[1,33] Approximately 1,000 cases of chancroid are diagnosed within the United States each year; the true incidence and prevalence of this disease is probably considerably higher.[6,33] Nevertheless, the low overall rates of chancroid suggest that it is a disease of limited communicability compared to trichomoniasis, gonorrhea, and syphilis.[52]

Infectious Etiological Agent

The etiological agent of chancroid known as the Ducrey bacillus (*Haemophilis ducreyi*) is a short, plump, gram-negative bacillus with rounded ends commonly observed in small clusters along strands of mucus, singly, or arranged in long parallel columns between cells or shreds of mucus.[12,33] Occasionally, the bacilli are situated intracellularly. The organism can be cultivated in whole defibrinated blood or nutrient broth containing blood; when grown in pure culture within a liquid medium, the Ducrey bacillus appears in long tangled chains composed of both coccal and bacillary (thus the term streptobacillus is often applied to this agent).[1,6,8,10,33]

Reservoir and Source of Infection

The reservoir is mankind. The source of infection is exudates (discharges) from open lesions and pus from buboes of patients; suggestive evidence exists that women may occasionally be carriers.[6] Chancroid is generally contracted via sexual intercourse, with lesions almost always located about the genitalia; the disease can be acquired from sexual partners who themselves show no clinical manifestations of chancroidal infection. The organism has been cultured from smegma and vaginal secretions from patients without discernable clinical disease.[33] Furthermore, organism readily produces an infection when inoculated upon open or abraded skin or mucous membranes.[6,33]

Mode of Transmission

Chancroid is generally transmitted by sexual or direct intimate contact except in rare instances of professionally acquired lesions upon the hands of physicians and nurses; accidental inoculation of children has been reported.[6] Prostitution, sexual promiscuity, and uncleanliness represent factors which favor transmission of this disease.[6,10] The disease may be transmitted by vaginal, anal, or oral-genital sexual contact, with bacteria most likely to invade the host at a point of existing injury such as a skin lesion or abrasion.[10] Nonsexual transmission of this disease appears to be most common in tropical regions.[6,10]

Incubation Period

The incubation period for chancroid is 1 to 5 days, generally 3 to 5 days.[6,10,33] Chancroidal lesions have been reported by some authorities to appear as early as 12 to 16 hours following inoculation.[17]

Period of Communicability

Chancroid is communicable as long as the infectious agent persists within the original lesion or discharging lymph nodes regionally; generally it parallels healing, and in most instances is a matter of several weeks.[6]

Susceptibility and Resistance

The susceptibility is general; there is no evidence of natural or acquired immunity.[6] Susceptibility to the disease appears greater within tropical regions.[33]

Signs and Symptoms

1. **Asymptomatic patients.** — Chancroid may present asymptomatically or simply as a mild vaginitis in females.[52]

2. **Lesions.** — When lesions develop, they most typically appear upon the labia, clitoris, fourchette, vestibule, anus, cervix, or penis.[17,52] The disease begins as an inflammatory macule that rapidly progresses to a vesicopustule to rupture and produce a nonindurated, shallow ulceration with an erythematous (red) margin.[52] The lesion is ragged and undermined with its base covered by a gray or yellow exudate.[52] Multiple lesions may develop, theoretically by autoinoculation. The lesions of chancroid are tender if not extremely painful, which provides some help in the differential diagnosis of syphilis; however, ulcerations upon the genitalia should always be subjected to Darkfield examination.[52]

3. **Lymphadenopathy.** — Inguinal lymphadenopathy develops in approximately 50 percent of patients, with chancroid within approximately 2 weeks of presenting skin lesions.[52] Satellite buboes are generally unilateral, with adenitis generally subsiding with gradual softening of the lymph nodes.[52] However, the nodes may suppurate and rupture.[1,33,52]

4. **Spontaneous regression.** — In rare instances, the lesions of chancroid may spontaneously regress even without treatment within a few days of their appearance.[6,10]

Presumptive Diagnosis*

Clinical Manifestations. — Generally a single but sometimes multiple development of superficial, painful ulceration surrounded by an erythematous halo. Ulcers may also be necrotic or severely erosive with ragged serpiginous borders. Accompanying lymphadenopathy is generally unilateral. A characteristic inguinal bubo occurs in 25 to 60 percent of patients; it may rupture. Ulcers generally occur upon the coronal sulcus, glans, or shaft; females are generally asymptomatic.

When the only organisms seen in a bubo aspirate or ulcer smear are

*From the Communicable Disease Center in Atlanta, Georgia.

arranged in chains or clumps along strands of mucus, and they are morphologically similar to *H. ducreyi*, the diagnosis is highly likely. A clinical presentation consistent with chancroid involving the genitalia and/or a unilateral bubo is suggestive. Since many STDs cause genital ulcers, it is crucial to differentiate them. All genital ulcerations should be examined by Darkfield microscopy.[12]

*Definitive Diagnosis**

The diagnosis becomes definitive when *H. ducreyi* is recovered by culture. Biopsy may be diagnostic but is not generally performed.[12]

*The Treatment of Chancroid**

1. Chemotherapy. — Erythromycin 500 mg p.o./q.i.d. or Trimethoprim/sulfamethoxazole, double strength tablet (160/800 mg) p.o./b.i.d. Chemotherapy should be continued for at least 10 days and until the lymph nodes and lesions have healed.

2. Lesion management. — Fluctuant lymph nodes should be aspirated through healthy adjacent normal skin. Incision and drainage or excision of the nodes will delay healing and is thus contraindicated. Compresses should be applied to the ulcers to remove necrotic material.

3. Additional measures. — The patient should return for reevaluation within 3 to 5 days following the beginning of chemotherapy. Sexual partners must be examined and treated as necessary. The patient should return weekly or biweekly for evaluation until the disease is cured. The prepuce should remain retracted during therapy, and the ulcerative lesions should be cleaned 3 times daily. However, retraction is contraindicated in the presence of preputial edema. Condoms should be utilized to help prevent future infections.[12]

---

*From the Communicable Disease Center in Atlanta, Georgia.

3. Condylomata Acuminata

Condylomata acuminata, or venereal warts, are common contagious benign epithelial tumors caused by a papovavirus. They generally present upon the skin and/or mucous membranes of the anogenital regions of both men and women.[1,11] The course of disease is erratic; infection may persist as a single lesion, or satellite lesions may develop by autoinoculation.[1] Complete regression may occur after months or years, with or without treatment; the appearance and size of the warts depend upon their location and the degree of irritation or physical trauma to which the warts are subjected.[1,33]

Occurrence

Mentioned in Greek erotic literature, "condylomata acuminata" literally means "knob" or "round tumor." The disease is common worldwide, with epidemic occurrences in families, dormitories, military bases, and institutions.[1,10,33] Venereal warts are the third and fourth most common form of STD for men and women respectively, with over 59,000 visits to physicians' offices alone each year (in the United States) for this condition.[14]

Infectious Etiological Agent

Warts are an infectious disease of the skin and contiguous mucous membranes due to a virus of the Papova group, which includes animal papilloma viruses, the polyoma, and simian vacuolating viruses, such as SV40 and SV5, which have been shown to induce tumors in experimental animals and to cause in vitro transformation of tissue cultures. The human wart virus is a DNA virus, measuring approximately 45 mu in diameter, which has been extracted from human lesions and has been utilized experimentally to induce the formation of warts at inoculated sites in the skin of human volunteers. Although the same virus is thought to cause all varieties of human warts, the character of the lesion itself depends upon the local response of the affected skin to the virus host. The virus has been

Condylomata Acuminata

shown electron-microscopically to parasitize the nuclei of epidermal cells. The skin lesions induced by the wart virus are due to an abnormal proliferation of epidermal cells. The lesions, which are skin-colored, may occur singly or in multiples widely disseminated over the entire body. The successful isolation of the human wart virus in tissue culture has not been accomplished conclusively.[33]

Reservoir and Source of Infection

The reservoir is mankind. The source of infection is contact with the virus generally, but not always by sexual contact.[16]

Mode of Transmission

The principal means of communication is sexual contact, but contraction of infection may occur by other means.[16] The probability of contracting the virus after sexual contact with an infected partner is estimated to be between 60 to 70 percent.[10,16,35] A study of 97 patients who had coitus with infected partners showed that 62 became similarly infected.[17] Transmission of infection is by vaginal, anal, and/or oral-genital sexual contact; however, warts have presented upon patients whose only sexual partner had no clinical manifestations of disease.[10] The warts may also be spread from one part of the body to another via autoinoculation.[1,10,16,17] Venereal warts in children may be a possible indication of child abuse.[62]

Incubation Period

The incubation period for venereal warts has been noted in studies to range from 3 weeks to 8 months, most commonly 1 to 3 months, with a mean incubation period of 2.8 months.[10,17]

Period of Communicability

The period of communicability is for the duration of the warts or presence of the virus.[1,10,16,17]

Susceptibility and Resistance

The susceptibility for this disease is general, with resistance to disease lowered by immune deficiency syndromes, stress, poor nutrition, lack of sleep, etc. Uncircumcised males are more apt to develop genital warts than circumcised males.[16]

Signs and Symptoms

1. Location of the warts may be single or multiple. In men, the warts tend to appear most commonly upon the glans, foreskin, urethral opening, penile shaft, and scrotum, in that order of frequency. In gay men, bisexual men, and women who have experienced rectal intercourse, the warts may be located around or within the anus. In women, most commonly the warts appear upon the bottom of the vaginal opening, but also occur upon the labia, and deep within the vaginal canal and endocervix.[16] Rare cases have been seen around the areola of the nipple in women, the margins of the mouth, and in the inguinal and axillary folds as well as in the interdigital skin regions between the toes.[33]

2. Appearance of the warts depends upon their location. Upon moist areas, the warts are generally pink or red and soft with a cauliflower-like appearance.[10] Multiple warts may grow together to form a very large tissue mass which can potentially obstruct the vaginal passage and/or rectal canal.[10,35] Upon dry skin, the warts tend to be small, hard, and yellow-gray, resembling ordinary skin warts appearing upon other parts of the body.[10,35] Genital warts tend to grow large if kept moist by vaginal and/or urethral discharges caused by such diseases as trichomoniasis, candidiasis, gonorrhea, NSU, etc.[10,35] For idiopathic (unknown) reasons, pregnancy can stimulate venereal warts to grow quite large.[10,35]

Presumptive Diagnosis*

A diagnosis can generally be made upon the basis of the typical clinical presentation. The physician should exclude the possible diagnosis of condylomata lata by obtaining a serologic test for syphilis.

Definitive Diagnosis*

A biopsy, although generally unnecessary, is required to make a definitive diagnosis. Very atypical lesions in which neoplasia is a concern should be biopsied before initiating therapy.[12]

The Treatment of Condylomata Acuminata*

1. Chemotherapy. — For small warts, Podophyllin (a dark red resin or oil from the mandrake plant) generally works quite well. The warts are first wiped clean utilizing a cotton applicator and a solution of 10 to 25

---

*From the Communicable Disease Center in Atlanta, Georgia.

percent Podophyllin is painted upon the warts, with lavage to follow within 1 to 4 hours to prevent a potential chemical burn.[10,35] The warts should dry up and fall off following one or several treatments. If the wart persists after 4 weekly applications, refer the patient to a dermatologist for liquid nitrogen therapy or electrosurgery. Note that Podophyllin should *not* be utilized during pregnancy or in instances of urethral or oral warts; most consultants recommend against its use for cervical or anorectal warts. Atypical or persistent warts should be biopsied. A Pap smear is recommended for all women with anogenital warts.[12]

2. **Alternative treatments** include cryotherapy (liquid nitrogen, solid carbon dioxide), electrosurgery, surgical removal (scissor or curette), and psychotherapy (hexing). *The Merck Manual of Diagnosis and Therapy*, as well as some dermatologists, notes that particularly with young children, suggestion accompanied by impressive but meaningless manipulations such as painting the lesions and exposing them to heat lamps is often remarkably successful in treating warts, but may be at least due to part to coincidental regression of the wart.[1,63]

3. **Control.**—Touching, scratching, and shaving warts can cause them to spread; an important part of treatment is the prevention of this kind of spread of these highly contagious lesions.[16,33,64]

4. Cytomegalovirus Infection (CMV)

Cytomegalovirus infection (CMV) is a sexually transmitted disease caused by the cytomegalovirus, which generally produces asymptomatic infection but may present as a nonspecific febrile illness, pneumonia, hepatitis, mononucleosis, or a combination of these.[12] Many authorities believe that cytomegalovirus infections may constitute the most important cause of birth defects such as mental retardation, blindness, and deafness.[29,30,66] In most adults there are few if any symptoms of infection, and the disease is of no great consequence except to pregnant women.[30]

Occurrence

A World Health Organization (WHO) scientific group meeting in 1979 estimated that approximately 1.5 percent of infants have congenital cytomegalovirus infection and that 15 percent of these infants suffer congenital defects.[14] Other investigators have stated that approximately one-half of all infants born to women with CMV infections contract the infection.[30]

Infectious Etiological Agent

The Communicable Disease Center in Atlanta, Georgia, has noted that CMV infections are due to the cytomegalovirus, a DNA virus of the herpes virus group.[12] The virus has been found in the cervix of women and in the seminal fluid of infected males.[29]

Reservoir and Source of Infection

The reservoir is mankind; the source of infection appears to be exudates from the endocervix and seminal fluid. The organism may also exist within saliva, urine, and feces, and may be transmitted sexually during intercourse.[29]

Mode of Transmission

It is currently believed that CMV infections may be transmitted via sexual intercourse and from the mother to her infant in approximately 50 percent of instances.[29,30] In one study, CMV was isolated from the cervix of 4.2 percent of 191 gynecological patients attending a general practice clinic and from 9.8 percent of 51 postpartum women attending the same clinic.[67]

Incubation Period

Idiopathic, but presumed to be similar to that of other virus-caused forms of sexually transmitted diseases.

Period of Communicability

A study in which the shedding of CMV was studied in 142 women who gave birth to congenitally infected infants showed that excretion of CMV was greater in younger women and fell to low levels by age 30.[68] Considering all sites of infection, 60 percent of the mothers of infected infants were shedding CMV within the first 3 months postpartum, compared with 18 percent of control mothers (N = 81); CMV shedding rates declined during the first 12 months postpartum to 35 percent in the former group and 3 percent in the latter. More than 3 years following delivery, 7 (15 percent) of 45 mothers who transmitted CMV still had the virus. The excretion of CMV is common and persistent in mothers of children with congenital malformations due to CMV infection.[68]

Susceptibility and Resistance

The susceptibility for this disease appears to be general. Studies have shown that CMV infection is an important variable affecting fetal outcome, with increased risk of intrauterine infection when the maternal infection occurs late in pregnancy; however, if fetal infection occurs earlier in pregnancy, it appears to present a greater threat to the fetus, with the potential for dissemination of virus in multiple fetal tissues, including the brain.[69]

Signs and Symptoms

The Communicable Disease Center in Atlanta, Georgia, notes that although generally asymptomatic, CMV infections may present as a nonspecific febrile illness, pneumonitis, hepatitis, mononucleosis, or a combination of these diseases.[12]

Presumptive Diagnosis*

Symptomatic contacts of definitively diagnosed CMV patients may be presumed to have CMV infection as well. Under unusual circumstances, this is a difficult diagnosis to establish, as CMV is associated with nonspecific clinical syndromes, and the diagnostic tests are very complex.[12]

Definitive Diagnosis*

Definitive diagnosis requires a rise in titer of the complement fixation (CF) or an immunofluorescent test in convalescent serum, or identification of the virus in tissues or secretions known to be previously negative in a symptomatic patient. Note that many healthy individuals shed CMV in their saliva, cervical secretions, urine, seminal fluid, breast milk, feces, and/or blood.[12]

Treatment*

Treatment is supportive, nonspecific and symptomatic; the disease is generally self-limiting among immunocompetent individuals. However, the acquired illness may provoke immunosuppression. Since it is not feasible to detect intermittent periods of infectiousness accurately at this time, no specific therapy is available, and there are no preventive measures other than utilization of a condom.[12]

---

*From the Communicable Disease Center in Atlanta, Georgia.

5. Enteric Infections

The Communicable Disease Center in Atlanta, Georgia, notes that enteric or intestinal infections may be caused by many bacteria, viruses, protozoa, and other organisms carried within the intestinal tract and may produce sexually transmitted disease. Such infections are typically asymptomatic or minimally symptomatic; symptomatic patients present with abdominal pain, abdominal cramping, diarrhea, nausea, and vomiting, all in highly variable degrees of severity. Many patients provide a history of frequent oral-genital and oral-anal sexual contact.[12] A study of 150 gay males in San Francisco revealed that 47 percent of the sample was positive for one or more potentially pathogenic intestinal protozoa.[70] *E. histolytica* was demonstrated in 54 (36 percent), *E. hartmanni* in 53 (35 percent), and *G. lamblia* in 7 (5 percent), with the prevalence of *E. histolytica* higher than that previously observed among gay men in other parts of the United States and Canada. Many of the men in the San Francisco study had more than one type of protozoan present; the most common combination was *E. histolytica, E. hartmanni,* and commensals.[70]

In an investigation of 89 sexually active gay males in New York, 23 (26 percent) harbored one or more protozoan pathogens; 18 (20 percent) showed *E. histolytica* infections; 11 (12 percent) had *G. lamblia*; and 6 (7 percent) were infected with both protozoa. Another study in New York involving 126 gay males revealed that 39.7 percent were infected with *E. histolytica* and/or *G. lamblia; E. histolytica* infected 39 (31 percent), while *G. lamblia* was demonstrated in 23 (18 percent).

Many investigators, then, feel that enteric sexually transmitted infections presently constitute a significant health threat to the gay, bisexual, and heterosexual population within the United States.[70]

Investigations have shown that the potential enteric pathogens include *Endamoeba histolytica, Endamoeba hartmanni, Dientamoeba fragilis, Giardia lamblia,* or any combination of these.[70] It should be noted that the pathogenicity of *Endamoeba hartmanni* remains controversial, while *Dientamoeba fragilis* was formerly considered to be nonpathogenic in nature.[8,70] Of the 150 gay males noted in the San Francisco study, of whom 71 (47 percent) had some form of potential pathogen, 70 percent were symptomatic.[70] While the practices of homosexuals particularly enhance enteric infections, Dritz and Goldsmith noted that oral-genital, oral-anal, and procto-genital sexual practices are not restricted to any single sector of the population or to individuals of specific sexual preference, thus placing heterosexuals at risk for these infections as well. However, Phillips and others have suggested that enteric parasites are less commonly found among heterosexuals as either there is an insufficient endemic rate or the number of sexual partners and prevalence of oral-anal sexual activity may be inadequate to maintain a sufficient level of exposure.[70]

Presumptive Diagnosis*

The typical clinical findings suggest enteric infection; a history of enteric infection in a recent sexual partner supports the diagnosis.

Definitive Diagnosis*

Definitive tests vary according to the involved agent: microscopic examination of ova and parasites for amebiasis and giardiasis; cultures for shigellosis; and serologic tests for hepatitis-A infections.

Amebiasis

Amebiasis, or amebic dysentery, is an infectious sexually transmitted disease caused by *Endamoeba histolytica*, producing a colitis characterized by the painful passage of bloody, mucoid stools but often causing only mild symptoms.[1] This large intestinal infection occurs in an asymptomatic carrier state in most individuals, but disease ranging from chronic, mild diarrhea to fulminant dysentery is frequently produced.[33] Among gastrointestinal complications, the commonest is hepatic abscess, which may rupture into the peritoneum, pleura, lung, and/or pericardium.[1,33] Infection is acquired via sexual contact or by ingesting of amebic cysts via food or drink contaminated by feces.[1] Infection may spread via the circulatory system or by direct extension to produce amebic hepatitis, abscess of the liver, lung, and brain, and/or ulceration of the skin. Amebiasis is an uncommon cause of death.[6]

Occurrence

Amebic dysentery constitutes a worldwide infection, often affecting 50 percent or more of populations within unsanitated areas, particularly

---

*From the Communicable Disease Center in Atlanta, Georgia.

within tropical countries and particularly within mental institutions.[6] The rate is low (1 to 5 percent) in well sanitated cities. Clinical amebic dysentery is most prevalent within warm and hot countries and relatively infrequent in temperate regions, although infection rates may be high and waterborne epidemics occasional.[6]

As a sexually transmitted disease, amebiasis has substantially increased in prevalence since the early 1970s within the United States, along with giardiasis and other forms of enteric infections.[70]

Infectious Etiological Agent

There are at least 6 different species of amoeba that parasitize the mouth and intestine of mankind. Principal among these is *Endamoeba histolytica*, which causes amebiasis and exists in two forms, the motile trophozoite and the nonmotile cyst.[33] The trophozoite is the parasitic form, generally 18 to 20 um in diameter (2.5 times the size of a red blood cell). It dwells within the intestinal lumen, divides by binary fission, grows best under anaerobic conditions, and requires the presence of either bacteria or tissue substrates to satisfy its nutritional requirements. It is capable of ingesting red blood cells when parasitizing the human organism.[8,33] The organism can be cultivated through several generations upon artificial laboratory media if these are properly enriched.[8]

The cyst is somewhat smaller than is the trophozoite, is rounded and nonmotile, and is more resistant than is the trophozoite to environmental pressures. When mature, it contains four nuclei, each capable of meiotic division, so that one cyst can give rise to eight trophozoites.[8] The cyst is highly resistant to environmental changes and is responsible for disease transmission.

Details of nuclear structure, cytoplasmic inclusions, and motility (in the case of the trophozoites) distinguish this organism from other forms of intestinal amoebas when they are microscopically examined.[8]

Endamoeba histolytica strains have been classified into large and small races depending upon whether they form cysts more or less than 10 u in diameter.[33] While it is possible that small strains (*E. hartmanni*) are less likely to produce symptoms than are the large strains, cyst size is apparently unstable, and the common statement that small strains are nonpathogenic is not justified.[33,70]

Endamoeba histolytica occurs normally within the intestines of a few dogs, monkeys, and rats; these animals, along with rabbits and kittens, can be infected experimentally.[33]

Reservoir and Source of Infection

The reservoir is mankind. The source of infection is infected human feces, which spread by direct oral-anal sexual activity or through contaminated food or water; water may be the source of epidemics.[8] Typically, the reservoir is a chronic or asymptomatic patient; acute disease is of little menace due to the fragility of the trophozoites (it is the cysts from the feces of infected persons that transmit disease).[6,8,33] An amebic disease in dogs occurs but has not been implicated as a source of human infection to date.[6]

Mode of Transmission

Amebiasis can be transmitted among both homosexuals and heterosexuals through oral-anal sexual contact.[70] Transmission is by sexual contact, water, food, hand-to-mouth transfer of fresh feces, contaminated vegetables (particuarly those served raw), and soiled hands of food handlers.[6,33] Epidemic spread is generally via sexual contact or contaminated water supplies, with extensive water-borne epidemics often due to contaminated, faulty hotel and factory plumbing. Where sanitary latrines are not utilized, flies and cockroaches may spread the cysts. The utilization of human feces for fertilization of growing vegetables and fruits, or the washing of foods in polluted water, leads to infection when the produce is eaten raw.[1]

Incubation Period

The incubation period for amebiasis is from 5 days to several months; commonly 3 to 4 weeks.[6]

Period of Communicability

The disease is communicable during the intestinal infection, which may continue for years.[6] The infective form of the parasite is the cyst, found in formed stools and capable when moist of existing outside the human organism at room temperature for 2 to 4 weeks.[1]

Susceptibility and Resistance

Susceptibility to infection is general. Relatively few persons harboring the organism develop clinically recognized disease; acute cases tend to become chronic.[6] Such infections appear to be particularly common to the gay and bisexual communities but may affect heterosexuals as well.[70] Malnutrition may contribute to the severity and frequency of this disease, with recent immigrants to endemic regions often contracting clinical disease. Immunity to reinfection has not been clearly established in mankind.[6] The factors responsible for ulceration extensive enough to cause symptoms are not clearly apparent; the size of the inoculation and the virulence of the infecting organism are both of significance, with bacterial flora of the intestine a potential major determinant of the extent of amebic disease. Germ-free animals cannot be infected with *E. histolytica* but become susceptible if the intestine is first allowed to acquire a normal complement of bacteria.[33]

Signs and Symptoms

Amebiasis is often asymptomatic; however, when "carriers" are treated, they realize that they have been experiencing mild symptoms related to this infection.

Gastrointestinal complaints are common; many patients, particularly in temperate climates, present with ill-defined gastrointestinal complaints of diarrhea, constipation, diarrhea alternating with constipation, fatigue, fever, vague somatic aches and pains, generalized or localized abdominal pain particularly within the right lower quadrant, and fatigue.[1,6] Infection may spread by the circulatory system or direct extension to produce amebic hepatitis; abscesses of the liver, lung, and brain; or ulcerations of the skin.[6] Some patients experience chronic diarrhea with mucus and blood.[6]

Symptoms diminish between relapses to recurrent cramps and loose or very soft stools due to colitis, yet emaciation and anemia tend to increase.[1]

Diagnosis

Marion Wilson, Ph.D., has noted the precise diagnostic methods for amebiasis:

Microscopic examination of feces is indicated when intestinal infection is suspected. Trophozoites remain active for a short time generally; thus stool specimens should be kept warm during their transport to the laboratory. Cold, casual specimens of stool are ordinarily not satisfactory for diagnosis of amebiasis. When chronic or asymptomatic amebiasis is suspected, mild purgatives are sometimes useful in increasing the concentration of cysts in stool specimens, thus facilitating laboratory diagnosis.

Aspirated pus from parenteral lesions or sputum may reveal the organisms when systemic localizations are suspected. Culture techniques are sometimes useful when microscopic examination fails to reveal the amoebae or cysts. Immunologic techniques are generally not completely dependable.[8]

Treatment

Dr. Wilson notes that tetracyclines are useful chemotherapy for intestinal amebiasis when combined with emetine. Arsenical drugs such as diodaquin or carbasone are also utilized. Parenteral abscesses may require surgical drainage. They are treated with quinine derivates such as chloroquine, coupled with antibiotics to control secondary bacterial infections.[8] Patients with amebic infections should be removed from food handling occupations until freed of the organism.

The Communicable Disease Center further notes that asymptomatic infected individuals for whom oral-anal sexual contact is a regular practice should be treated as symptomatic patients, as should those most readily able to transmit the disease (food handlers, hospital workers, day care employees, etc.). The patient should avoid oral-anal sexual contact at least until the infection is cleared; sexual partners should be referred for diagnosis and treatment, with an early return for additional treatment if symptoms become persistent or recur.[12]

Cryptosporidiosis

Cryptosporidiosis is similar to amebiasis and may be responsible for many cases of "untreatable" diarrhea, particularly among homosexuals. The symptoms include anorexia, low-grade fever, abdominal cramps, and 5 to 10 watery/frothy bowel movements per day, followed by constipation. Diagnosis is by testing stool specimens for oocysts of cryptosporidium utilizing the Sheather's sugar-flotation technique. Like some forms of dysentery, this disease is self-limiting in immunologically healthy individuals, disappearing within several weeks. Little is known concerning the treatment of this rare human disease (most commonly found in sheep, deer, and cattle), and for those with immunodeficiency, it may represent a serious and life-threatening disease.[73]

Giardiasis

Giardiasis (also Lambliasis, G. intestinalis, Lamblia intestinalis, Giardia lamblia, or Giardia) is a potentially sexually transmitted disease of the intestinal tract due to *Giardia lamblia*.

Occurrence

Kean has directed considerable attention to the problem of both amebiasis and giardiasis as significant sexually transmitted diseases. The homosexual population is at particular risk for such infections, which may affect heterosexuals as well.[70] As the sexual practices of gay and bisexual males enhance fecal-oral contamination in some instances, gay and bisexual males constitute a population at risk for this disease.[70]

Infectious Etiological Agent

Giardia lamblia is a pear-shaped, multiflagellar, protozoan parasite (subphylum Mastigophora) with two developmental stages. It possesses two nuclei, which give the organism the appearance of a face with two eyes when viewed microscopically.[8,33] Residing within the human duodenum, the parasite can invade the intestinal mucosa.

The two developmental stages of *Giardia lamblia* consist first of a trophozoite stage, which has a tumbling, vibrant motility imparted by several pairs of flagellae located upon one side of the pear-shaped body as well as a pair of symmetrically located nuclei, which resemble eyes or spectacles. The trophozoite is approximately twice the size of a red blood cell in length and approximately half this in diameter. In contrast, the cyst stage is the infectious stage of the disease, with the cyst a nonmotile, oval shaped structure with 4 nuclei when mature. Flagellar protoplasts can be seen within the cytoplasm.[8]

Reservoir and Source of Infection

The reservoir for giardiasis is mankind; the source of infection is infected human feces.[8,33] The infective form is the cysts from direct contacts. The organism ordinarily resides saprophytically within the duodenum and jejunum asymptomatically but produces clinical manifestations of disease when the organism reaches sufficient numbers to involve large surface areas of the large intestine.[8]

Mode of Transmission

The source of infection is infected cysts within human feces, which may be transmitted during oral-anal sexual practices or other forms of fecal-oral contamination.[8,33,70]

Incubation Period

The incubation period is similar to that for amebiasis, 5 days to several months; most commonly 3 to 4 weeks with many patients remaining asymptomatic.[8,33] One recent study of 150 gay patients in San Francisco revealed that 70 percent were symptomatic.[33,70]

Period of Communicability

The disease is communicable while the intestinal infection persists — potentially for years.[8]

Susceptibility and Resistance

Susceptibility is general, with many patients asymptomatically harboring the organism within the intestinal tract.[8] The population at risk is the gay and bisexual communities, with heterosexual individuals, particularly those engaging in oral-anal sexual activity, at particular risk as well.[70] Children are 3 times more likely to be parasitized than are adults, and children tend to have more prominent clinical manifestations of disease. (See *Signs and Symptoms*, below). The response to infestation is highly variable and related at least in part to host factors. Gastrectomy or decreased gastric acidity in adults may increase their susceptibility to giardiasis, which is also more frequently reported in patients with immunoglobulin deficiencies.[33]

Signs and Symptoms

Most commonly, patients are asymptomatic for this infection.[8] Symptomatic patients typically present with nausea, vomiting, flatulence, epigastric pain, abdominal distention, weight loss, and watery diarrhea. These symptoms are more commonly seen in children and are generally self-limited.[33] Rarely, fulminating and extensive duodenal ulceration occurs.[8,33] Pale stools may be seen, along with dehydration.[8]

Diagnosis

The diagnosis is based upon clinical manifestations of disease and laboratory tests, with the presence of giardiasis in a recent sexual partner supportive of the diagnosis.[12] Definitive diagnosis is by microscopic demonstration of the organisms in duodenal washings, jejunal biopsies, or diarrheal stools.[33] Cyst forms containing 2 to 4 nuclei are often passed and may be readily identified when stained with iodine.[8,33]

Treatment

The treatment consists of administration of 0.1 gm of Atabrine hydrochloride 3 times daily for 3 days, a regimen which eliminates the parasites in 90 percent of patients.[33] Metronidazole (Flagyl) 250 mg 2 times a day for 5 to 7 days has also been shown to be effective.[33] Oral-anal sexual contact should be avoided until the infection has cleared; sexual partners must be referred for evaluation and treatment; and the patient should return early if symptoms persist or recur.[12]

Complications and sequelae vary with the disease agent, health of the host, therapy, and many other factors in instances of enteric infection.[12] Spontaneous cures are common; yet morbidity in other cases may be severe, requiring hospitalization and intravenous hydration.[12] Infections may become systemic, with chronic giardiasis leading to malabsorption and pathogenesis which is still not completely understood. Jejunal biopsy of patients infected with giardiasis sometimes shows flattening of the microvilli and an inflammatory infiltrate.[33]

Shigellosis

Shigellosis, or bacillary dysentery, is an acute, self-limited, infectious disease restricted to the intestinal tract. Shigellosis is considered to be a sexually transmitted enteric disease.[12]

Occurrence

Shigellosis occurs in all parts of the world. In tropical and subtropical populations of underdeveloped countries, shigellosis is a frequent and serious disease, occurring at all ages and responsible for many deaths.[6] The disease is most frequent within jails, institutions for children, and mental hospitals.[6,33] Within the United States, shigellosis is endemic in lower socioeconomic regions and upon Indian reservations, with occasional epidemics, mainly in the warmer seasons.[6] As a sexually transmitted disease, shigellosis is most common among those engaged in oral-anal contact with a wide variety of sexual partners.[6]

Infectious Etiological Agent

There are 27 serotypes of the genus *Shigella* (dysentery bacillus) currently recognized, which are in 4 main groups: Group A — *Sh. dysenteriae*; Group B — *Sh. flexneri*; Group C — *Sh. boydii*; and Group D — *Sh. sonnei*, with serotypes of each.[6] In epidemics and endemically, more than one serotype is commonly present and cases not infrequently show mixed infection with other intestinal pathogens.[6] *Shigella* organisms are nonmotile, nonencapsulated, slender, gram-negative bacilli which may appear as coccobacilli upon initial isolation.[33] They are aerobes of facultative anaerobes which grow best at 37°C; they have rather simple nutritional requirements and have the ability to grow in the presence of bile salts.[33]

Reservoir and Source of Infection

The reservoir is mankind; the source is feces from a carrier.[6,8,33]

Mode of Transmission

By direct contact via fecal-oral transmission, or indirectly by objects soiled with feces or by eating contaminated foods or drinking contaminated water or milk.[6] Flies which have fed upon human feces may spread the infection as well.[6,33] Contaminated food or water is responsible for the widest distribution of the disease.[8]

Incubation Period

The incubation period may range from 1 to 7 days.[6,33]

Period of Communicability

The disease is communicable during acute infection and until the organisms are absent from feces, generally within a few weeks.[6,33] The carrier state does not develop so frequently in shigellosis as it does in salmonellosis; rarely, the carrier state may persist for 1 to 2 years.[6,8]

Susceptibility and Resistance

Susceptibility is general, but the disease is more common and more severe in children than in adults.[6] Another population at risk is those engaged in frequent oral-anal sexual activity with a large variety of sexual partners.[70] The disease is more common in countries lacking adequate sanitation and in institutions, with the disease extremely rare during the first month of life. Studies of volunteers have shown that it is necessary to ingest very large numbers of the bacilli to establish infection within mankind.[33] Concerning immunity, specific antibodies develop during the course of the disease but are not protective against new infections.[8]

Signs and Symptoms

Sudden onset in younger children is typical, with fever, irritability, drowsiness, anorexia, nausea, vomiting, diarrhea, abdominal pain, abdominal distention, and tenesmus (rectal spasm making defecation difficult). Within 3 days, pus, blood, and mucus appear within the stools, and the stools often increase to 20 or more per day, with weight loss and severe dehydration often present. An untreated child may die within the first 12 days; if the patient survives, acute symptoms generally subside within the second week.[1]

Enteric Infections

Adult clinical manifestations are largely afebrile, with nonbloody and nonmucous diarrhea and little or no tenesmus; however, onset in some adults is characterized by griping abdominal pain, urgency to defecate and passage of formed feces initially, which temporarily relieves the pain. These episodes occur with increasing severity and frequency; diarrhea becomes marked, with soft or liquid stools containing mucus, pus, and blood. The disease often resolves spontaneously within 4 to 8 days for mild cases and 3 to 6 weeks for severe cases.[1]

It should be noted that mild diarrhea or asymptomatic infections are not uncommon in instances of shigellosis. Hyperactivity of bowel sounds is common; convulsions are most common in children.[33] Splenomegaly has been reported but is rare.[1,33]

Diagnosis

Diagnosis of shigellosis is facilitated by a high index of suspicion during outbreaks, particularly within epidemic regions; however, the disease cannot be distinguished from salmonella gastroenteritis except through identification of the etiological agent.[1,39] Differential diagnosis should include ulcerative colitis, nonspecific or viral diarrhea, celiac sprue, cholera, amebiasis, intestinal parasites, and infantile *E. coli* diarrhea.[1,8,24,71]

Definitive diagnosis involves the isolation of Shigella from stool samples. Smears should be examined for parasites, blood, and pus; agglutinins develop too irregularly to be of diagnostic significance.[1,8]

Treatment

1. Fluid therapy. — Dysentery generally causes isotonic dehydration. Excessive water intake can cause hypotonicity. In infants, dehydration may cause hypertonic serum. Premature administration of high-solute fluids (milk, tube feedings, "homemade" electrolyte mixtures) may cause damaging hypertonicity, including convulsions.[1]

2. Antibiotics. — With proper fluid replacement, antibiotics are often unnecessary, and resistance to them is now widespread, varying with the species. *S. sonnei* isolates are likely to be resistant to ampicillin and tetracycline, but oxolinic acid 20 mg/kg/day in 2 doses at 12 hour intervals (for adults) given for 5 days is effective. Despite resistance to tetracycline, successful therapy has been achieved by administering it in a bolus of 3 gm over a half-hour period (in adults). Trimethoprim with sulfamethoxazole (as for typhoid fever) will eradicate organisms quickly from the intestine. Ampicillin 3 gm/day for 5 days will cure most *S. flexneri* infections.[1]

3. Other treatment. — Anticholinergics and paregoric should be avoided. The patient's progress should be carefully followed until the stools are consistently free of Shigella.[1]

Gonococcal Disease

There are four main kinds of gonococcal disease:[1,2,6,8]

- *Gonorrhea of columnar and transitional epithelium* —this includes mucous membrane infections of gonococcal origin including gonococcal urethritis, gonococcal cervicitis, gonococcal pharyngitis, and gonococcal proctitis.
- *Gonococcal vulvovaginitis of female children* —an inflammatory reaction of the urogenital tract of prepubescent females characterized by erythema (redness) and edema (swelling) of the mucous membranes associated with varying degrees of mucopurulent urethral exudate (mucus-pus discharge). It is a self-limited disease; more than 75 percent of patients recover spontaneously within three to six months, although a carrier state may sometimes persist.[6]
- *Gonococcal ophthalmia neonatorum* —acute gonococcal infection of a neonate's (newborn's) eyes with erythema (redness), edema (swelling) of the conjunctiva of one or both eyes, mucopurulent or purulent discharge, and ultimate blindness within several days if untreated by prophylactic or therapeutic measures (required in all states at the time of birth).
- *Metastatic Gonorrhea* —this includes gonococcal septicemia, gonococcal dermatitis, gonococcal arthritis, gonococcal salpingitis, and adult gonococcal conjunctivitis. This represents gonococcal infections of the circulatory system, skin, joints, fallopian tubes, and eye respectively.

Gonorrhea of Columnar and Transitional Epithelium

Gonorrhea of columnar and transitional epithelium differs in males and females with respect to the course of the disease, its seriousness, ease of identification, and response to therapeutic measures, along with degree of infectivity.[1,6]

Common names for gonorrhea include *clap, gleet, dose, strain, running rage, drip, morning drip* and others. Essentially, the word "gonorrhea" means "flow of seed" and was named such by Galen, a Greek physician, in A.D. 130.

History

Gonorrhea is probably the oldest and definitely the most prevalent reported communicable disease in the United States today. It appears that the first record of the disease was upon Egyptian tablets dated 3500 B.C. while Chinese writings mention the disease in 2637 B.C. The book of Leviticus in the Bible mentions the disease (dating back perhaps to 1500 B.C.).[10,16,17]

Hippocrates in 400 B.C. believed that gonorrhea resulted from "excessive indulgence in the pleasures of Venus" (the Roman goddess of Love) while Galen mistakenly believed that the infection arose from an "involuntary loss of male seminal fluid".[10,16,17]

In A.D. 1161, brothels in London were forbidden to house prostitutes suffering from the perilous infirmity of burning (the burning paid of urination or dysuria), while the French called gonorrhea "hot piss" and introduced the slang term "clap" for the disease in the 1300s.[10] During the Middle Ages, gonorrhea and syphilis were believed to be the same disease, which set back scientific progress in understanding and curing these diseases: an English physician, Dr. John Hunter, inoculated himself with bacteria from a gonorrhea patient but unfortunately, the patient also had syphilis and Dr. Hunter developed the symptomatology associated with both diseases.[16] Thus, the mistaken conclusion was that gonorrhea and syphilis were in fact, the same diseases. In 1793, the French General Carnot wrote that venereal diseases transmitted by the 1,300 prostitutes serving his soldiers "killed 10 times more men than enemy fire!"[10] In 1830, syphilis and gonorrhea were distinguished as separate diseases by Philip Ricord, although it was in 1879 that Dr. Albert Neisser identified the bacteria (named after him) which causes the disease (*Neisseria gonorrhoeae*); in 1943, it was noted that penicillin constituted an effective treatment of this disease.[16,17] This led to a de-emphasis on previously energetic venereal disease control programs with contact-tracing no longer considered to be of particular significance.[7] The first significant gonorrhea epidemic occurred after World War I; the incidence declined in the 1930s and then rose again during World War II to levels as high or higher than today.[10] With the end of war and the development of penicillin, the rates declined to an all-time low in the 1950s.[10] The downward trend in gonorrhea incidence reversed itself in 1959; a 1968 survey indicated that physicians were treating 80 percent of diagnosed syphilis and gonorrhea but were reporting only one-fifth of these cases.[7] While gonorrhea was initially easily treated, today "super gon" or the new drug resistant forms of gonorrhea which have been apparent in some states since early 1977, largely arising from self-treatment among prostitutes in Vietnam, continue to make the ultimate control of gonorrhea much more difficult.[10,17]

Occurrence

Gonorrhea is still probably the most common communicable disease in the U.S.; over one million cases are reported each year with an estimated four million actual cases of gonorrhea.[9,13,14,16,17,20] Worldwide, some authorities note that there may be as many as 150 million cases of gonorrhea, many of which remain undiagnosed and untreated.[7] From 1975 until 1984, the disease has shown a slight but significant decline[16] which may be due to two factors: the National Gonorrhea Control program and changes in treatment.[16,17,18]

By 1979 teenagers were engaging in sexual activity with a greater frequency and at an earlier age than they had in the early 1970s.[19] Reported gonorrhea among teenagers within the U.S. peaked just over 250,000 cases in 1981 with approximately 60 percent of all patients females.[19] Over the past two decades, older teenagers had persistently higher gonorrhea rates than did younger teenagers.[19] Currently, the diagnosis of gonorrhea among teenagers is more prevalent than the diagnosis in childhood of varicella (chicken pox), which is the fourth most common communicable disease reported within the U.S.[16,19] The most prevalent age group for gonorrhea within the U.S. presently is 20 to 24 years, with rates higher in urban than in rural areas.[16] Alaska has the highest gonorrhea rate and Vermont has the lowest; San Francisco has the highest gonorrhea rate of any major city within the United States.[16] Until 1945, GC ranked third among the reported communicable diseases, following measles and syphilis.[20] Beginning in 1946, syphilis and gonorrhea switched ranks and since 1965 gonorrhea has been the most common reported communicable disease within the U.S.[20]

The Pennsylvania Department of Health has noted that some 600 or more cases of gonorrhea have been traced to a single person and that some 11-year-old children have reported over 32 sexual contacts upon seeking treatment.[21] The Department reveals that "core transmitters" are often largely responsible for spreading gonococcal infection; a group of 323 women with gonorrhea, for example, were found to have had spread the infection to 1,008 male sexual partners.[16] This means over three sexual contacts per woman in this instance as compared with 0.92 sexual contacts per infected person nationally.[16,22] Some people attending STD clinics for treatment have reported that they have had over 1,000 different sexual contacts in one year.[23]

Etiological Agent

The etiological agent for all forms of gonorrhea is the same, *Neisseria gonorrhoeae*, which is a bean-shaped, gram-negative, intracellular diplococcus bacterium.[1,8,9] Because the agent is morphologically indistinguishable from the meningococcus, it cannot be identified by morphological characteristics alone in stained smears of purulent exudates; gram-negative diplococci other than the gonococcus may cause infections of mucosal tissue either alone or in conjunction with gonorrheal infection.

Generally, the organism dies quickly outside of the human body; however, a study by Gilbaugh and Fuchs in 1979 revealed that gonococci placed upon a toilet seat or upon paper remained viable enough to cause infection of another individual up to two hours later. Within a moist environment such as upon a towel, these bacteria may remain viable for up to 24 hours.[16] Combs has noted that the gonococcus in another study was shown to remain viable for eight hours and that it is a "sturdier" organism than is the syphilitic spirochete, *Treponema pallidium*.[13]

Although in physical appearance and staining characteristics, the gonococcus is the very image of the meningococcus, that is where the similarity ends.[24] The gonococcus in culture is more difficult to grow; when allowed to dry it generally dies immediately; it is a complete parasite living on a human host; and it does not reside within the human organism as a harmless commensal.[24] In view of such characteristics, it is somewhat surprising that the gonococcus manages to hold "its place" in the natural world, but that it does succeed is only too evident.[24]

Reservoir and Source of Infection

Mankind is the only reservoir of gonococcal infections; the organism does not remain viable in "subhuman animals" although the chimpanzee shows promise in studies to develop a vaccine (probably the only ultimate control measure for the disease) at the University of Pittsburgh Medical Center.[6,25] The source of infection is typically exudates (discharges) from the mucous membrances of an infected host.[1,6,10,16] Studies have revealed an extremely high STD rate among gay males but an insignificant incidence among gay females. Only three percent of infected males name another male as the infectious contact; 12 to 18 percent of syphilitic males name another male as the reservoir of infection. Unger found that the same STDs which occur in gay people occur also in heterosexuals, although the site of infection is often different.[17] Heterosexual males typically develop gonococcal urethritis, while gay males may develop gonococcal proctitis along with urethritis and pharyngeal infection. The probability of infectivity for pharyngeal infection is estimated at 5 to 10 percent for cunnilingus versus 20 to 30 percent for fellatio.[10]

Mode of Transmission

Gonorrhea is transmitted almost entirely by direct sexual contact, even in children. It is occasionally transmitted to the newborn in the form of an ophthalmic infection during passage through the vaginal canal and, in institutions, to children by the careless and indiscriminate utilization of rectal thermometers.[1,6] The principal means of communication is genital-to-genital contact; it may also be spread by oral-to-genital and anal-to-genital contact. The probability of acquiring infectivity during genital-to-genital contact is approximately 20 to 50 percent—often specified by medical authorities as approximately a "one in three chance." That is, nationally, one-third of those individuals who have sexual intercourse with an infected patient infect themselves.[10,16,22] During fellatio, females, gay, and bisexual males have an approximately 10 to 20 percent chance of infectivity; whereas in the case of cunnilingus, gay females and heterosexual and bisexual males have an approximate five to ten percent chance of infection.[10,16,22] A study of U.S. Navy personnel in the Philippines revealed that without the use of a condom, the risk of infectivity by male-to-female sexual intercourse is approximately 20 to 30 percent after one or two sexual acts.[16] There is evidence that the infection may spread in females from the vaginal canal into the rectum; however, many women, when specifically questioned, admit to having rectal intercourse for birth control purposes, sexual pleasure, or both.[10,16] Approximately 10 to 20 percent of males with gonococcal urethritis are asymptomatic compared to ranges of 15 to 90 percent for gonococcal cervicitis (often noted to be 75 to 90 percent) and 70 percent in the instance of rectal infection, although severe symptoms may evidence themselves for rectal and for pharyngeal gonorrhea, which is often asymptomatic as well.[10,16] Women using birth control pills may increase their degree of infectivity from 20-30 percent to virtually 100 percent. The pill discourages the use of condoms and vaginal contraceptives, which make the infection less likely, and causes a pH change within the vaginal tissues themselves, making a "foothold" for such infection much more probable.[10,16,17] Fomite transfer of gonorrhea (by nonliving objects) for the most part is highly unlikely unless objects contaminated with fresh infectious discharges come into direct contact with the genital or conjunctival mucosal tissues.[1,7,8]

Incubation Period

The incubation period for gonorrhea is three to four days generally, with a range of from one to 31 days following infectivity.[1,6,10,16,17] In the instance of ophthalmia neonatorum, the incubation period is generally 36 to 48 hours.[1,6,8] Again, it must be recognized that asymptomatic infections are particularly common in instances of gonococcal proctitis, pharyngitis, and cervicitis.[1,6,9,16,17] It must also be recognized that the nature of the signs and symptoms themselves change with time as in the instance of mucopurulent urethral exudate or dysuria in the male.[1,6,8,16]

Period of Communicability or Infectivity

Communicability is for months or years unless the infection is definitively treated by chemotherapy; most of the gonococci die within two to nine hours, and signs and symptoms of the infection are relieved generally within two to three days.[10,16,17] Following treatment, the patient may be noninfectious within 24 hours but must not be assumed to be so until several days have passed and until a follow-up culture is performed approximately one week following diagnosis and treatment.[1,10,16] In the instance of vulvovaginitis in young females, the disease generally does not persist for more than six months, while infected conjunctival membranes should be considered so until all exudate discharge has ceased.[1,8]

Susceptibility and Resistance

Susceptibility is general without respect to age, sex, race, and reinfection may readily occur.[1,6,8] Spontaneous recovery is typical in the absence of reinfection.[6] Effective natural immunity to gonorrhea, thus, most definitely does not develop as a result of infection, and artificial immunization is not available at this time.[1,8] A vaccine developed at the University of Pittsburgh Medical Center is being refined but is not ready for use.[25] The utilization of a condom and/or birth control foam may reduce the chance of infectivity by 80 percent.[23] The probability for infectivity varies greatly with the site of infection.

Signs and Symptoms: Males — Gonococcal Urethritis

1. The appearance of a thick mucopurulent urethral exudate (mucous/pus discharge) from the penis generally three to nine days postinfection with a potential range report of from one to 30 days (most commonly within three to four days).[1,8,16,17,23,26] This exudate typically is white but may be a yellow or yellow-greenish color which comprises dead urethral cells, pus (dead white blood cells), and live white blood cells as the gonococcus is highly toxic to the mucosal tissues of the urethra.[1,10,23] The exudate may be initially light and become heavy, disappearing within two weeks postinfection if treatment is not sought, then spreading upward to create potential complications.[1,8,10,16] This discharge may be atypically present only in the morning.[10,23]

2. Dysuria and frequency of urination. — Severe dysuria or severe urinary pain which initiates at the urinary meatus and spreads throughout the shaft of the penis is typical; in addition there is typically frequency of urination, which is associated not only with gonococcal urethritis but with gonococcal prostatic infections as well. In the case of prostatic infection, there may be difficulty initiating a urinary stream as well as weak or interrupted flow of urine. There may also be difficulty stopping the flow of urine. In addition, the urine may be hazy and contain some blood (hematuria).[1,8,10,23] Hematuria is most common following 10 days without treatment.[10]

3. Potential inguinal lymphadenopathy.—Approximately 30 to 40 percent of males with gonococcal urethritis experience inguinal lymphadenopathy or regional lymphadenitis, an enlargement of the lymph nodes of the groin along the inguinal crest of the thigh. In severe instances there may be satellite buboes or matted lymph nodes.[1,10,23]

4. Erythema and edema of the urinary meatus.—Typically, there is erythema (redness) and edema (swelling) of the anterior meatus (end of the penis), with periurethral abscess (infection circumferentially around the penis) most frequently in uncircumcised males.[1,6,8,10,23]

5. Untreated, the infection spreads upward in the urethra toward the prostate gland, seminal vesicles, bladder, epididymis, and inguinal lymph nodes, and may enter the circulatory system (gonococcal septicemia) to cause metastatic gonorrhea of the following forms: gonococcal dermatitis, gonococcal arthritis, and other systemic infections in the male.[1,10,16] Inflammation of the heart and spine are particularly severe complications which affect approximately one to three percent of all gonorrhea patients.

After about two weeks without treatment, the dysuria and exudate disappear. Approximately five to ten percent of males then develop a prostatic abscess, causing feelings of heat, edema, and pain within the lower quadrants of the abdominal cavity and urinary difficulty and frequency due to prostatic hypertrophy (infectious enlargement of the prostate). It may be impossible to urinate until treatment is sought or the abscess ruptures, releasing infectious pus exudate into the penis and/or rectum.[10]

Periodically, males with such infections may evidence a return to more obvious signs and symptoms such as dysuria and mucopurulent or purulent exudate (pus discharge).[1,8,10,23] Approximately 20 percent of males untreated for a duration of one month develop infections of the vas deferens and the epididymis. Probably due to a circulation difference, gonococcal epididymitis most frequently occurs on the left testicle.[10] Gonococcal epididymitis presents as pain within the groin, a heavy sensation upon the affected testicle.[1,8,10,23] The skin overlying the scrotum may become red, warm, and painful.[1,10,23] Gonococcal epididymitis leaves scar tissue which may partially or totally obstruct the passage of seminal fluid containing sperm from the affected testicle, and the formation of a hard and painful edema on the bottom of the affected testicle.[1,8,10,23] Fortunately, as gonococcal epididymitis is generally unilateral sterility does not typically result.[1,6,8,10,23] However, untreated, the unilateral infection may become a bilateral gonococcal epididymitis, resulting in sterility. But even with delayed treatment, total recovery is the rule.[1,8,10,16,17]

6. **Atypically, gonococcal urethritis may be asymptomatic or subclinical.** It is presently estimated that approximately 10 to 26 percent of all males with gonococcal urethritis are asymptomatic or subclinical (without discernible signs and symptoms).[10,17,23] It is possible for one to be an asymptomatic carrier and transmitter of gonococcal infection.[1,8,23] However, studies by Ginsberg (1980), Handsfield (1974), and Taub (1976) have revealed that gonococcal urethritis tends to be symptomatic in approximately 80 to 90 percent of infected males. The dysuria largely arises from mucosal damage in contact with uric acid, as well as potential stricture of the urethra arising from repeated and particularly severe infections characteristic of certain strains of *Neisseria gonorrhoeae*.[1,8,10,17] Urethral stricture may require surgical treatment.[1,7,8] Rosen (1972) noted some atypical signs and symptoms of GC infection such as primary infection of the penile skin and gonorrhea-induced infection of accessory genital glands.[27,28]

7. **Slight malaise and slight hyperpyrexia.** — Fatigue and a slight fever may arise from gonococcal infections.[29]

Signs and Symptoms: Females — Gonococcal Cervicitis

1. **Females are generally asymptomatic.** Approximately 50 to 90 percent of females are asymptomatic for gonococcal cervicitis, generally specified at 80 percent.[7,16,17,30,31] The columnar epithelium of the cervix represents the most frequent site of infection in women.[1,10,31] A major symptom of gonorrheal infection in women is a gonococcal infection in her male sexual partner, who needs to inform her of the possibility of a GC cervical infection.[1,16,17]

2. **Dysuria** is an infrequent symptom, as the female urethra is apt to be less severely infected than in the male.[1,10,31] Severe symptoms from gonococcal urethritis in the female sometimes develop and include dysuria, frequency of urination, and a mucopurulent urethral exudate, which may be expressed by "milking" the urethra with digital pressure.[1,10,31]

3. **Vaginal discharge.** — Some women experience a vaginal discharge due to gonococcal cervicitis; however, this discharge is typically slight and often goes unrecognized.[1,10,31] For this reason, some medical authorities believe that some 640,000 or more women may have gonorrhea without knowing it.[7,10,31]

4. **Edema of the Bartholin glands, malaise, and slight hyperpyrexia** may result in some women; untreated, approximately 30 to 50 percent of women develop such Bartholin gland infections (deep within the labia majora).[10,16,17] In approximately one to two percent of infections, one gland becomes edematous and painful with a slight exudate.[10,21]

5. Low backache and vague pain within the lower abdominal quadrants is seen in some instances of gonococcal cervicitis.[1,10,17]

6. Trichomonal vaginalis vaginitis infection may arise in conjunction with gonococcal cervicitis infections for unknown reasons in approximately 50 percent of instances.[1,10,31] The symptoms for this potential infection include an abundant frothy yellow-green vaginal exudate; erythema (redness), pain, and severe pruritus (itching), making walking, sexual intercourse, and sleeping painful if not impossible; a distinctive "mushroom-like" odor arising from the genitalia; and inguinal lymphadenopathy (enlarged lymph nodes within the groin).

7. Gonococcal Proctitis. — GC rectal infections are seen in approximately 40 to 60 percent of women with gonococcal cervicitis, with approximately 70 percent of cases asymptomatic.[10,17] In some cases, the proctitis results in nonspecific signs and symptoms such as diarrhea, severe burning pain on defecation, a sense of incomplete evacuation of the bowel, blood and pus exudate in the stool, and abdominal pain.[1,10,17]

8. Pelvic Inflammatory Disease. — In approximately 50 percent of untreated women, the gonococcal infection enters the uterus within approximately eight to ten weeks.[1,10,17] *Neisseria gonorrhoeae* does not readily survive within the endometrium except during menstruation, when bacteria can multiply within the dead endometrial cells (one bacterium can multiply into 68 billion within approximately 12 hours, while 2 billion bacteria may be contained within a single drop of water, exudate, urine, feces, saliva, seminal fluid, etc.).[10,32] During menstruation, the infection spreads readily into the fallopian tubes, causing gonococcal salpingitis (PID), a form of metastatic gonorrhea in which pus exudate leaks from the fallopian tubes into the pelvic cavity and onto the ovaries themselves.[1,8,9,10] The fallopian tubes can be blocked; should this occur bilaterally, sterility may arise. (An estimated 80,000 women per year are rendered sterile by gonococcal salpingitis.[10,30]) Should the infection be either unilateral or bilateral in a recently fertilized female, an ectopic pregnancy may arise in which the fertilized egg becomes trapped within the fallopian tube due to obstruction of passage associated with the infection.[1,10,17,33] Even following chemotherapy with antibiotics, 20 to 30 percent of women with gonococcal salpingitis have tubes which will remain blocked. The typical signs and symptoms of gonococcal salpingitis are:

A. A longer and more painful menstrual period.
B. Severe pain bilaterally within the lower abdominal quadrants.
C. Nausea, vomiting, and fever over 102°F.
D. There may be pain during sexual intercourse.
E. There may be abnormal vaginal bleeding due to the disruption of hormonal secretions (when the ovaries are seriously affected by infection).

F. Subacute salpingitis may be difficult to diagnose, as symptoms are mild and may be caused by a variety of other gynecological disorders such as appendicitis, ectopic pregnancy, etc. Sometimes, exploratory surgery is essential to make a definitive diagnosis and provide definitive treatment. Some infected women may suffer from a gonococcal pelvic residue resulting in repeated infections; such women usually require hysterectomy to stop the cycle of infection.[1,7,8,10,13,34]

Benjamin Kogan notes that approximately 50 percent of hospital patients with fallopian tube infections have gonococcal salpingitis.[7] Furthermore, eighty percent of patients with gonococcal arthritis and other forms of disseminated gonococcal infection are women.[7] Probably 12 percent of all asymptomatic females with gonorrhea (75 to 90 percent of the total case load) develop pelvic inflammatory disease.[7]

Gonococcal Pharyngitis and Tonsillitis

The human oral mucosa appears to be more resistant to *Neisseria gonorrhoeae* than to *Treponema pallidum*, which causes syphilis; by far the predominance of gonococcal infections involve the urinary tract.[7] Nonetheless, gonococcal pharyngitis and tonsillitis are commonly seen in STD clinics, particularly within urban areas with large gay male populations.[7,10] Gonococcal pharyngitis is rarely reported from kissing and cunnilingus; generally it arises from fellatio.[1,10,23]

A study by Owen and others involving 11 patients with gonococcal pharyngitis revealed that this infection was symptomatic in only three patients (approximately 25 percent), who evidenced typical pharyngitis symptomology such as pharyngeal pain, erythema (redness), and exudate discharge. There may be tonsillitis, peritonsilar abscess, and/or cervical lymphadenopathy. Seven of these eleven patients were cured with 4.8 million units of APPG, or 3 gm. tetracycline hydrochloride taken orally by those with penicillin allergies. That gonorrhea can be transmitted from the oral mucosa to the penis appears evident from military personnel who have contracted gonococcal urethritis from fellatio by prostitutes.[1,10,23]

The incubation period for gonococcal pharyngitis and tonsillitis appears to be generally one to two days postinfection for those who become symptomatic; such patients not infrequently have gonococcal or other STD infections elsewhere within their bodies. Metastatic gonorrhea involving gonococcal septicemia, dermatitis, and arthritis has been reported from primary pharyngeal infections of gonorrhea.[7] The normal Cowper's glands secretions discharged from the penis prior to ejaculation should not be confused with an infectious exudate.[35]

Gonococcal Proctitis

Gonorrheal infection of the rectum is seen in gay and bisexual males and in heterosexual females and is asymptomatic approximately 70 percent of the time.[17] Owen's study of 19 patients with gonococcal proctitis confirms other statistics that rectal GC infections tend to present vague signs and symptoms if any at all. Eight of his patients were asymptomatic. Symptoms reported among the others included rectal itching (four patients), rectal fullness (three), bloody discharge (three), diarrhea (three), mucus discharge (two), rectal pain (one), rectal hemorrhoids (one), rectal chafing (one), and rectal warts (one).[33] Some patients in this study complained of pain during defecation.

Thus, when signs and symptoms of gonococcal proctitis do appear they are often associated with factors other than the infection, such as the trauma of vigorous rectal intercourse, irritating substances utilized as lubricants, and/or other medical problems unassociated with the infection itself.[1,10,23]

Pariser noted that 62 of 307 females with positive rectal cultures for gonococcal proctitis acknowledged having rectal sexual intercourse. Other investigations have noted that at least 75 percent of women with gonococcal proctitis have had rectal sexual intercourse.[37,38] Elaborate theories to otherwise explain gonococcal proctitis, such as migration of an infectious agent from the vaginal to the rectal canal or contamination via the medium of a rectal thermometer, are given less validity today.[10,32]

Gonococcal Vulvovaginitis of Female Children

Gonococcal vulvovaginitis of female children represents a gonococcal inflammatory reaction of the urogenital mucosa of prepubescent females, more superficial in nature than adult vulvovaginitis and characterized by erythema (redness), mucous membrane edema (swelling), mucopurulent exudate (mucous/pus discharge) of varying degrees, and in severe infections, excoriation (abrasion of tissue) of the labia and thighs and extension to urethra and bladder.[1,6] It is a self-limited disease; 75 percent or more of all patients spontaneously recover within three to six months, although a carrier state may sometimes persist.[1,6,33]

Identification

Gonococcal vulvovaginitis is to be differentially diagnosed of acute vulvovaginitis due to other etiological agents; in the USA, approximately 25 percent of all vaginitis is gonococcal.[6] Some forms of vaginitis cannot be distinguished definitively by clinical manifestations alone; rather, diagnosis is by bacteriologic culture of exudates, as stained smears are not completely reliable.[1,6,33] Authorities disagree on the extent to which gonococcal vulvovaginitis results from contact with fomites.[1,6,24,32] Within an exudate discharge, the gonococcus may survive under favorable conditions outside of the human organism for up to 24 hours.[13,16,17]

Occurrence

Epidemics occur frequently in institutions for females.[6] The full extent of this disease is idiopathic (unknown) but presumably worldwide and widespread.[6] Individuals with poor personal hygiene habits and/or early and frequent sexual activity are prone to this disease. Transient and inapparent infections may exist among children.[6]

Infectious Etiological Agent

Neisseria gonorrhoeae.

Reservoir and Source of Infection and Mode of Transmission

Infection is through sexual or other forms of intimate direct contact with infected adults.[6,8] The source of the infection is exudates (discharges) from the infected host; infrequently, contaminated and moist articles.[6,8] The existence of transient inapparent gonococcal infection among children has been demonstrated.[6]

Incubation Period

Generally three to nine days.

The Period of Communicability

The disease is communicable while the exudate (discharge) persists—generally three to six months—and, in some instances, after the disappearance of clinical manifestations of disease.[6,8]

Susceptibility and Resistance

Susceptibility or degree of potential infectivity is dependent upon the type of epithelium lining the vaginal canal. Until puberty it is columnar or transitional epithelium; after puberty, it is stratified squamous epithelium which is not attacked by *Neisseria gonorrhoeae*.[6,8] The susceptibility is general for female children; the frequency of spontaneous recovery indicates a developing resistance.[1,6,8] An infection of gonococcal vulvovaginitis does not provide an immunity against future infections.[6,8,10,36]

Recommended Control Methods for Gonococcal Vulvovaginitis*

Preventive measures are fundamentally dependent upon the control and eventual eradication of gonorrhea as well as proper hygienic measures within homes and institutions to prevent fomite-induced infections.[6,8]

Control Measures

- Report to local health authorities, required in most states by law.
- Isolation — For 24 hours following administration of chemotherapy.
- Quarantine — None.
- Specific Treatment — Penicillin in a single repository dose.
- Concurrent disinfection — Caution in the disposal of materials contaminated with exudate discharges for 24 hours or longer.
- Immunization of contacts — None. Chemotherapy is provided upon suspicion of infection.
- Investigation of contacts — Check for sexual and other forms of child abuse.

Gonococcal Ophthalmia Neonatorum

Gonococcal ophthalmia neonatorum, conjunctivitis neonatorum or acute conjunctivitis of the newborn, represents a purulent conjunctivitis of the neonate's eyes acquired at birth during passage through the gonococcally infected vaginal canal.[1,6,8] There are other types of nongonococcal infections which may arise from etiological agents such as staphylococci, streptococci, pneumococci, meningococci, hemophilic bacilli, and bedsonial microorganisms.[1,6,8,23]

Occurrence

Occurence is worldwide but varies considerably depending upon the preventive measures taken or legally required at birth within various

---

*From the American Public Health Association.

localities. It is infrequent where prophylactic measures are taken to treat a potential gonococcal infection at birth with either one percent silver nitrate solution or penicillin drops.[1,10,33] Many obstetricians prefer penicillin drops to silver nitrate as they now believe that penicillin provides better antibiotic protection and generally results in less conjunctival irritation.[1,10] Better yet is to treat the mother prior to delivery when possible; studies within the United States and Canada reveal that approximately five percent of pregnant women have gonococcal cervicitis.[10] Globally, the disease still represents a significant cause of blindness.[6,8]

Infectious Etiological Agent

Neisseria gonorrhoeae.

Reservoir and Source of Infection and Mode of Transmission

Mankind represents the only reservoir of infection; the source of the infection is gonococcal mucopurulent vaginal exudate in direct contact with the neonate's conjunctiva during passage through the vaginal canal at birth.[1,6,8,10,17]

Incubation Period

In gonorrheal infections of the neonate's eyes, signs and symptoms generally appear within 12 to 48 hours (but up to four days) after birth.[1,6,8,33] Inflammation of the conjunctiva with vaginal gonococcal exudate is rapidly followed by erythema, edema, pain, and purulent exudate, with eyes swollen shut and the occurrence of blindness within a few days without definitive treatment.[1,6,8,10,17] Furthermore, there may be chemosis (edema of the conjunctiva about the cornea), lid edema, and bulbar infection of the lids.[1,2,6,8]

Period of Communicability

Communicability lasts until the gonococcal exudates from infected conjunctiva cease (approximately 24 hours following definitive therapy).[1,6,8]

Diagnosis

Clinical manifestations of severe conjunctivitis are characterized by erythema, edema, purulent exudate, eyes swollen shut, chemosis, bulbar infection, and/or edema of the eyelids along with gram-stained scrapings from the retrotarsal fold in the newborn evidencing conjunctivitis.[1,6] Gonococci are generally readily apparent upon a gram stain of the purulent exudate, and if treatment is instituted early, results are quite favorable.[1,10,33]

Treatment

Both systemic and topical antimicrobial chemotherapy prevent the spread of infection to the unaffected eye as the disease is generally unilateral initially.[1,33] The conjunctival sac should be frequently irrigated with normal saline solution (.9 percent sodium chloride solution – N.S.S.) to prevent secretions from adhering to the eye; the pupils should be kept dilated with atropine sulfate if there is corneal involvement.[1,33] Irrigations should be continued until all evidence of exudate (discharge) has disappeared.[1,10,33] All purulent inflammations of the conjunctiva should be regarded as gonococcal until proven otherwise.[6,10,33]

Prognosis

Excellent with immediate definitive treatment.[1,33]

Prophylaxis

Routinely instilling two drops of one percent silver nitrate solution (soln) into each eye immediately after birth has tremendously reduced the incidence and prevalence of blindness due to this disease.[1,6,10] Infrequently, this procedure will cause a sterile (chemical) conjunctivitis, but it should be performed as this disease still results in blindness to significant extent throughout the world.[6] Expectant mothers with gonorrhea must be treated during pregnancy and prophylactic treatment given to all infants at birth.[1,33]

Control Measures

- Prophylactic treatment of the neonate's eyes at birth required in most states.
- Depends upon the eradication of gonorrhea ultimately.
- Report to local health authorities.
- Health education activities.
- Isolation – For the first 24 hours after chemotherapy.
- Concurrent disinfection – Caution in the disposal of contaminated articles with exudate discharge.
- Endemic measures – None.

Metastatic Gonorrhea or Disseminated Gonococcal Infections (DGI)

With the increasing numbers of individuals who develop acute gonorrhea each year, the complications of disseminated gonococcal infections (DGI) are also being seen more frequently.[23,31] This is particularly true for females, who are generally 75 to 90 percent asymptomatic for gonococcal cervicitis, as well as for an individual with pharyngeal or rectal gonorrhea, both largely asymptomatic.[1,6,7,8,10,23,33]

In approximately one to three percent of all cases of untreated gonococcal infection, the gonococcus within a few weeks spreads from the mucous membrane tissues of the pharynx, rectum, vagina, or penis into the circulatory system causing gonococcal septicemia or gonococcemia, which in turn provides for further metastasis into bone tissue (gonococcal arthritis), skin tissue (gonococcal dermatitis), conjunctival tissue of the adult eye (adult gonococcal conjunctivitis), fallopian tubes (gonococcal salpingitis) as well as other organs and tissues throughout the human organism.[1,10,31]

Complications arising from metastatic gonorrhea or disseminated gonococcal infections are classified as either local or distant.[9,31] Local complications include:

Females	Males
• Involvement of Skene and Bartholin glands	• Phimosis-paraphimosis
	• Periurethral abscess
• Parametritis	• Involvement of glands of Tyson, Littre, and Cowper
• Cystitis-trigonitis	
• Proctitis	
• Pelvic inflammatory disease (PID) (Salpingitis, pelvic abscess, pyosalpinx, adhesions, peritonitis, tubo-ovarian cyst)	• Prostatitis
	• Seminal vesiculitis
	• Epididymitis
	• Trigonitis
	• Stricture
• Sterility	• Sterility

Distant complications may develop either by direct inoculation, as in the eye, pharynx, or rectum, or via metastatic spread within the human organism to the heart, brain, or joints. Rarely in adults is adult gonococcal conjunctivitis contracted via infectious exudate upon fingers or fomites.[1,10,31] Hematogenous metastasis of the gonococcus in the form of a true gonococcemia can lead to the involvement of many organs for which cutaneous lesions may be the only symptomology (gonococcal dermatitis, which is temporary).[1,10,31] The skin lesions generally begin as discrete erythematous papules which rapidly progress to a vesiculopustular stage; purpura or hemorrhagic bullae may develop.[31,33]

Hopefully, the early diagnosis and treatment of acute gonorrhea will prevent the development of these metastatic complications and their severe sequelae. The distant complications of gonorrhea include the following:[31]

- Meningitis
- Pharyngitis
- Pneumonia
- Septicemia
- Arthritis
- Tenosynovitis
- Bursitis
- Periostitis
- Conjunctivitis
- Panophthalmitis blindness
- Myocarditis, endocarditis, pericarditis
- Proctitis*
- Cutaneous lesions

A pregnant woman inflicted with gonorrhea is at higher risk in general for spontaneous abortion, prematurity, and stillbirth.[1,10,23]

Gonococcal Septicemia or Gonococcemia

Gonococcal septicemia or gonococcemia (gonorrheal infection of the circulatory system or bloodstream) is much more common in females and gay or bisexual males in whom gonorrheal infections tend to be asymptomatic.[1,8,16,17] In approximately 65 to 75 percent of gonococcemia patients, the following signs and symptoms present themselves:[1,10]

- Fever — 100 to 104°F
- Chills
- Anorexia (lost appetite)
- Generalized fatigue and feeling of ill health
- Polyarthritis — Joint pain in more than one joint, or migratory polyarthritis in which the pain migrates from joint to joint. The joints most commonly affected are the knees, wrists, fingers, hands, ankles, and elbows in that order.[10,33]

Very rarely, gonococcemia produces a febrile illness which is so similar to meningococcemia that differentiation upon clinical manifestations alone is impossible.[1,33]

Endocarditis due to gonococcemia has virtually disappeared due to the effective chemotherapeutic agents now available to treat gonorrhea prior to metastasis.[33] Left-sided endocarditis with the involvement of the aortic valve is the most common form of endocarditis seen today; however, the gonococcus "favors" the tricuspid and pulmonic valves as well.[33] In addition to petechiae, glomerulonephritis, embolic phenomena,

---

*May represent primary site of involvement.

anemia, and splenomegaly, two clinical features of gonococcal endocarditis may suggest the diagnosis. Jaundice, presumabely due to "toxic" hepatitis, is very common, and the majority of patients have two distinct spikes of fever during a 24-hour period (the double quotidian pattern).[33]

Gonococcal Dermatitis

In approximately 50 percent of gonococcal septicemia patients, a characteristic gonococcal dermatitis presents, characterized by a skin rash upon the arms, hands, legs, and feet, particularly around joints.[1,10,33] At first, a pinpoint erythemic (red) spot appears, which quickly becomes raised and blister-like with slight bleeding.[1,10,31] The center of the lesion then becomes pitted and grayish in color with an irregular violet border surrounding it.[1,10,31]

Gonococcal dermatitis is slightly painful, unlike the syphilitic secondary rash, and healing occurs within three to four days, leaving a faint dark spot.[1,10] Within approximately four to five days, the bacteria within the circulatory system die, and symptoms of gonococcal dermatitis disappear.[10]

Gonococcal Arthritis

An acute arthritis can result from the invasion of joints by *Neisseria gonorrhoeae*, generally associated with a past or present infection of gonococcal urethritis, cervicitis, proctitis, or pharyngitis.[1,10,33]

Occurrence

Arthritis occurs as a manifestation of gonococcemia in approximately one percent of patients. In the past, it primarily occurred in males and destroyed the involved joints; today it is seen predominately in females and gay or bisexual males.[1,10,31,33] If treated early, gonococcal arthritis responds well to antibiotic chemotherapy, leaving no residual joint damage.[33] Gonococcal arthritis has largely passed into the realm of the forgotten due to immediate definitive therapy of gonorrhea and rarely, gonococcal arthritis when it occurs.[24]

Infectious Etiological Agent

Neisseria gonorrhoeae.

Incubation Period

Symptoms appear within seven to ten days of the initiation of gonococcemia. Particularly in females and gay or bisexual males, the infection may follow an exacerbation of an indolent or subclinical infection.[1,33] The onset is often abrupt, with a clinical picture of fever, arthralgia, and painful arthritis.[1,10,33]

Signs and Symptoms

In 50 percent of patients, the characteristic gonococcal dermatitis appears prior to the appearance of the arthritis, generally upon the distal portion of the extremities or around joints.

In 80 percent of instances, gonococcal arthritis is polyarticular; the knee is the most frequently involved joint, followed in order of frequency by wrists, ankles, hands, elbows, hips, and shoulders.[1,10,33]

Tenosynovitis occurs in 50 to 75 percent of cases, and should call attention to the potential gonococcal infection.[33]

Polyarthritis and tenosynovitis similar to rheumatic fever are followed by joint suppuration (pus formation), with the knee, wrist, and ankle being the most frequently affected joints.[1] The joints are hot, erythemic, exquisitely tender, painful on motion, contain excessive fluid, and appear baggy due to localized edema. Typically, there is a history of primary gonococcal infection which was asymptomatic or untreated.[1,10,33]

Diagnosis

Acute arthritis in a patient with gonococcal infection strongly suggests the potential for gonococcal arthritis.[1,10,33] Arthrocentesis (joint aspiration) with smear and culture of the aspirated fluid along with the history and clinical manifestations of disease establish the diagnosis.[1,33] Careful bacteriologic study of joint fluid often fails to reveal gonococci, particularly if patients are seen relatively early in the course of this disease.[33] Loss of joint space due to the destruction of cartilage appears rather quickly upon x-rays.[1]

Treatment

Penicillin represents the most preferred specific treatment and should be given IM in dosages of 1.2 million units or more every six hours for 10 to 14 days, with the joint aspirated daily to provide drainage and prevent permanent damage.[1,33] Intra-articular penicillin is not recommended by medical authorities.[1]

Penicillin is so effective in treating gonococcal arthritis that poor therapeutic response to large dosages of penicillin casts serious doubt upon the diagnosis itself.[1] Joint symptoms generally begin to improve within a few days of treatment, and complete recovery occurs within one to two weeks.[33] In an occasional patient, however, the response to treatment is less dramatic, with the persistence of symptomology for a much longer period of time.[33] Completely penicillin-resistant agents for gonococcal arthritis have not been isolated as yet; reported instances have represented misdiagnosis, reinfection, and/or inadequate penicillin therapy.[1]

Gonococcal Salpingitis or Pelvic Inflammatory Disease

As stated in the discussion of gonococcal cervicitis, following eight to ten weeks without treatment, approximately 50 percent of patients develop gonococcal salpingitis or pelvic inflammatory disease (the less-preferred term) representing a form of metastatic gonorrhea.[1,6,10,33] The infection can lead to obstruction of the fallopian tubes leading to sterility, ectopic pregnancy, and many other types of complications.[1,33] Symptoms include a longer/more painful menstrual period, severe pain bilaterally within the lower abdominal quadrants, nausea, vomiting, hyperpyrexia (over 102°F), painful sexual intercourse, and abnormal vaginal bleeding. Signs and symptoms often disappear following one to two weeks of bed rest.[1,7,8,10,13,34] Salpingitis is the most frequent and serious complications of gonococcal cervicitis in women.[17]

Adult Gonococcal Conjunctivitis

Adult Gonococcal Conjunctivitis is a rare but severe purulent conjunctivitis in adults due to *Neisseria gonorrhoeae* (the gonococcus), generally acquired via the medium of self-inoculation (direct contact to the eye) with gonococcal exudate from a genital infection, contaminated fingers, or freshly soiled articles.[1,33]

Occurrence

Worldwide, but less frequent today than in the past because of the emphasis upon the treatment of pregnant women infected with gonococcal cervicitis or vaginitis and the precautions taken in the management of exudates from infected patients.[1,6]

Infectious Etiological Agent

Neisseria gonorrhoeae.

Incubation Period

The disease becomes apparent generally within 12 to 48 hours following inoculation of the conjunctiva with infectious gonococcal exudate.[1,6]

Signs and Symptoms

Generally, the condition is initially unilateral (affecting one eye). The clinical manifestations of disease are similar to but more severe than gonococcal ophthalmia neonatorum (conjunctivitis neonatorum), and complications, including corneal ulcerations, abscesses, perforations, panophthalmitis (inflammation of the entire eye), and blindness are more common in the adult form of the disease.[1,8]

Reservoir and Source of Infection

The reservoir is mankind only; the source of infection is gonococcal exudate which comes into contact with the conjunctiva of the adult eye.

Mode of Transmission

Adult gonococcal conjunctivitis may be acquired by people of all ages, generally via the transfer of genital infection by contaminated hands.[1,8,10] Patients and medical personnel may infect themselves in this manner if they are careless about hand washing following contact with a gonococcal exudate or should some of the exudate contact the adult eye of medical personnel during delivery of infants.[1,8]

Treatment

The treatment is essentially the same as for conjunctivitis neonatorum (gonococcal ophthalmia neonatorum) but with more emphasis upon parenteral antimicrobial chemotherapy along with topical therapy to prevent blindness.

Control Measures

- Report to local health authorities.
- The control and eventual eradication of gonorrhea; treatment of pregnant women for gonorrhea prior to delivery.
- Definitive treatment of mother and infant after birth when treatment cannot be provided prior to birth in rare instances.
- Washing of hands following contact with exudate; avoidance of touching anything following contact with the exudate.
- Isolation—None.
- Contact tracing—None.
- International measures—None specific other than the control and eventual eradication of gonorrhea.
- Quarantine—None.
- Immunization of contacts—None.
- Concurrent disinfection—Caution in the disposal of articles contaminated with exudate discharge.
- Epidemic measures—None; a sporadic (rare) disease.
- Specific treatment—Parenteral penicillin; one percent tetracycline solution or oily suspension may be applied locally as an adjunct to safeguard against penicillin resistance.

Prophylaxis

The best agent for prophylaxis following contact of the conjunctiva with gonococcal exudate has not been definitively determined. One percent silver nitrate solution may be superior to penicillin G; other medical authorities believe that penicillin drops provide better antibiotic protection with less irritation.[10,33]

Miscellaneous Complications of DGI

Gonococcal Amniotic Infection Syndrome

Within the past decade, it has been determined that the gonococcus may infect a pregnant woman's uterus, resulting in premature birth, premature rupture of the amniotic sac (24 hours prior to delivery), inflammation of the umbilical cord, and maternal fever.[7] It has not been conclusively proven that this form of metastatic gonorrhea is the exclusive cause of this condition; however, it is known that pregnant women with untreated gonorrhea experience higher rates of a variety of obstetrical complications, including stillbirth.[1,7,10,23,33]

Urethral Stricture

The gonococcus is highly toxic to the mucosal tissues of the urethra; untreated urethritis or repeated infections of gonococcal urethritis may lead to fibrosis and urethral stricture, making urination difficult and masking the typical signs and symptoms of gonococcal urethritis.[1,24]

Reiter's Syndrome

Gonococcal infections may be associated with Reiter's syndrome, a disease or idiopathic etiology characterized by urethritis, conjunctivitis, and polyarthritis, generally in that order. The conjunctivitis is nongonococcal in nature and a PPLO (pleural-pneumonialike organism) may be the infectious etiological agent.[1] Gonorrhea responds to appropriate antibiotic chemotherapy; Reiter's syndrome persists.[1]

Gonococcal Epididymitis

A painful and serious complication of untreated gonococcal urethritis is gonococcal epididymitis, characterized by edema of the maturation chamber connecting the testes and vas deferens.[1,2] The testes may become as large as oranges (orchitis) and extremely painful due to the infection.[17]

Pyelonephritis

Untreated gonococcal urethritis may metastasize to the kidney, with kidney damage possible. Metastatic gonococcal complications such as this frequently result in symptoms such as malaise, marked debility, fever, and abdominal pain. Such complications repeatedly caused the death of gonorrhea patients prior to the advent of antibiotic chemotherapeutic agents.[17]

The Diagnosis of Gonorrhea*

Presumptive Diagnosis
(warrants full treatment and follow-up)

Microscopic identification of typical gram-negative intracellular diplococci on a smear of urethral exudate (men) or endocervical material

---

*Information from the Communicable Disease Center in Atlanta, Georgia, unless otherwise noted.

(women); *or* growth on selective medium demonstrating typical colonial morphology, positive oxidase reaction, and typical gram-stain morphology.

Definitive Diagnosis

Growth on selective medium demonstrating typical colonial morphology, positive oxidase reaction, typical gram-stain morphology, and confirmed by sugar utilization, coagulation or antigonococcal fluorescent antibody (FA) testing. A definitive diagnosis is required if the specimen is extragenital, from an infant or child, or of medicolegal significance.[9,12]

Diagnosis — Men

Recommended Criteria

1. Microscopic demonstration of gram-negative intracellular diplococci on a smear of urethral exudate constitutes sufficient basis for the diagnosis of gonorrhea. The smear should be preprared by rolling the swab upon the slide; otherwise microscopic morphology will be distorted. If positive, treat for gonorrhea; if negative, culture for *N. gonorrhoeae* and treat the patient for nonspecific nongonococcal urethritis (NGU).[9,39]

2. Culture specimen — When gram-negative intracellular diplococci cannot be identified upon a direct smear of urethral exudate, a culture specimen should be obtained from the anterior urethra and innoculated upon Thayer-Martin (TM) or Transgrow medium. The combination of a positive oxidase reaction of colonies and gram-negative diplococci grown on either medium provides sufficient criteria for a definitive diagnosis of gonorrhea.

3. Test of cure — When a test of cure or a test for incubating gonorrhea is needed, a culture specimen should be obtained from the anterior urethra and plated upon either medium; the culture should be interpreted according to the combination of criteria presented in item 2.

4. Gay and bisexual males — An additional culture specimen should be obtained from the pharynx and rectum and inoculated upon TM or Transgrow medium, and interpreted as in item 2.

5. Clinical examination — If the male is not circumcised, the physician should pull back the foreskin with a gloved hand, checking for lesions and exudate discharge as well as dysuria and edema. Each testicle is gently squeezed to check for gonococcal epididymitis (this aspect of the examination should be painless unless such infection is present). The groin should be examined for inguinal lymphadenopathy (enlarged lymph nodes) and upon finding such, the patient should be checked for generalized lymphadenopathy syndrome (GLS). The patient's temperature should be taken as well as the patient's history of sexual contact. Often the diagnosis of gonorrhea is apparent upon clinical examination; however, definitive diagnosis by laboratory tests is always indicated.

6. **Techniques not recommended:**
    A. Fluorescent antibody staining of smears of urethral exudates is not recommended to diagnose gonorrhea.
    B. Fluorescent antibody staining of urethral exudates or the delayed fluorescent antibody procedure should not be utilized as a test for cure.[9,12]

7. **Patient follow-up** — The patient should be instructed to return to the clinic or physician's office within one week of the initial visit for cultures to establish a cure or to provide further definitive treatment as needed.

8. **Patient failure to respond to chemotherapy:**
    A. Check for compliance with medication or evidence of "milking" urethra.
    B. Repeat gram stain and culture for *N. gonorrhoeae*.
    C. Do wet prep for trichomoniasis; if the sexual partner has trichomoniasis, treat the patient for this even if the wet prep is negative.[39]
    D. Do a gram stain for candida.
    E. Consider rarer causes such as urinary tract infections, etc.[39]
    F. Every gonorrhea patient should receive a VDRL or RPR for syphilis.

9. **Lesions** — Consider and test for the following conditions:
    A. Condylomata accuminata
    B. Granuloma inguinale
    C. Ulcerative — Rule out trauma.
        (1) Syphilis — Perform darkfield exam.
        (2) Chancroid — Perform gram stain and culture.
        (3) Herpes — Typical lesions allow for a presumptive diagnosis; a Pap or Tzanck smear may be helpful; culture is the most sensitive and most specific test if specimen is obtained from an unbroken vesicle.[39]
    D. Balanitis — Erythema, plaques, exudate. May be nonspecific or due to gonorrhea, trichomoniasis, or candida. The diagnosis should be made as described under item 1.

Gonococcal Disease

   E. Condylomata lata — Perform darkfield exam.
   F. Molluscum contagiosum.

10. **Inguinal lymphadenopathy:**
   A. Search for genital lesions and proceed as per lesions, above.
   B. Consider granuloma inguinale, lymphogranuloma venereum, AIDS, and generalized lymphadenopathy syndrome.
   C. Examination for generalized lymphadenopathy as evidence of GLS or other systemic infections.

11. **Potential proctitis infection** — Approximately 70 percent of gonococcal proctitis cases are asymptomatic; itching, bloody discharge, constipation, diarrhea, and rectal pain are noted as the most common symptoms. Kogan notes that itching represents the single most common symptom.
   A. Perform gram stain for *N. gonorrhoeae*. If positive, treat for gonococcal proctitis and obtain culture.
   B. If work-up for gonorrhea is negative, do a serology for LGV, rule out syphilis, and consider other causes, particularly in gay males, such as giardiasis, amebiasis, shigella, chlamydia, and other pathogens; refer the patient for further GI work-up.[39]

12. **Contacts** — Defined as male patients whose sexual partners have been definitively diagnosed as having one or more specific infections.[39]
   A. *Syphilis* — Thorough examination, history, RPR, cultures; treat patient as for primary syphilis for contact within 90 days.
   B. *Gonorrhea* — Thorough examination, history, RPR, smear and cultures; treat patient as for uncomplicated gonorrhea for contact within 30 days.
   C. *Trichomonal vaginalis vaginitis* — Thorough examination, history, RPR, smear and culture; treat the patient as for this infection. If the infection does not respond, consider treatment for other forms of vaginitis which respond to different chemotherapy.[10]
   D. *Enteric pathogens* — Refer for further GI work-up.

13. **Epididymo-orchitis** — Defined as painful, tender, swollen testes and/or gonococcal epididymitis.[39]
   A. Perform a urinalysis and urine culture and sensitivity.
   B. Do a urethral smear and cultures for gonorrhea and for chlamydia (if available).
   C. Rule out torsion (surgical emergency), trauma, etc.

14. **Miscellaneous medical information of importance concerning the diagnosis of gonorrhea and its differential diagnosis:**
   A. Every STD patient should have complete cultures for gon-

orrhea and an RPR serologic test for syphilis (which diagnoses 70 percent of primary syphilis patients, many of whom do not recall a primary lesion.[10,39]

B. Noninfective dermatologic conditions affecting the penis are generally benign but may be malignant. Cancer of the penis is more common in uncircumcised and Chinese males.[40] Benign lesions include sebaceous cysts, seborrheic keratoses, benign papillomata, vitiligo, lichen planus, psoriasis, eczema, contact dermatitis, fixed drug eruption, and pearly penile papules. Malignant lesions and premalignant lesions include balanitis, xerotica obliterans, lichen sclerosis et atrophicus, erythroplasis of Queyrat, leukoplakia, squamous cell carcinoma, Kaposi's sarcoma, mycosis fungoides, melanoma.[39] Thus, dermatologic consultation may be required for any unusual or nonhealing lesions and is strongly suggested.

C. If the darkfield examination is negative and follow-up highly likely, the patient may be reevaluated without treatment. Repeat RPR and an FTA-ABS are indicated along with reevaluation within one week. Then, if the RPR and FTA-ABS and darkfield examinations are negative, the patient should return within one month for another RPR and FTA-ABS. If negative, the RPR and FTA-ABS should be repeated within two months.[39] A positive RPR should be confirmed with an FTA-ABS; however, when syphilis is likely clinically, treatment should not be delayed while awaiting the results of the FTA-ABS.[39]

The Diagnosis of Gonorrhea in Men — Summary

Acute gonococcal urethritis is readily diagnosed in males as the clinical course of disease is highly suggestive and bacteriological confirmation can be quickly established. While a positive gram stain can confirm the presence of gonorrhea, a negative gram stain *does not* rule out gonococcal infections. If the gram stain is negative, culture evidence may be obtained by taking a specimen from the anterior urethra. Suspected gonococcal pharyngitis and proctitis may be confirmed by culture examination of the pharynx and rectum respectively.[31] For the rectal culture, a sterile cotton-tipped swab is inserted approximately one inch into the anal canal allowing several seconds to allow for absorption of exudate. If the swab is inadvertently pushed into feces, another swab is utilized for the culture.[31]

Complications of Gonorrhea in Men — Summary

Men are at risk for epididymitis, sterility, prostatitis, urethral stricture, and infertility.[9,12]

All gonococcally infected individuals untreated are at risk for metastatic gonorrhea or disseminated gonococcal infection (DGI) including gonococcal septicemia (gonococcemia), gonococcal dermatitis, gonococcal arthritis, gonococcal meningitis, and gonococcal endocarditis, as well as adult gonococcal conjunctivitis.[1,10,12,33]

Diagnosis — Women

Recommended Criteria

1. Culture specimens and gram stain from endocervix — Cultures of the pharynx and rectum should be taken and an RPR and/or FTA-ABS performed.[1,10,39] Culture specimens are inoculated upon separate Thayer-Martin (TM) culture plates or in separate Transgrow bottles. The combination of a positive oxidase reaction of colonies and gram-negative diplococci grown on either medium provides sufficient criteria for at least a presumptive diagnosis of gonorrhea (gonorrhea exists but there may be other infections as well).[39]

2. Test of cure — Culture specimens should be obtained from the endocervix, rectum, pharynx, and urethral canal and inoculated on either TM or Transgrow medium, and interpreted according to the combination of criteria present in item 1.[9,12]

3. Techniques not recommended:
   A. Gram-stained or fluorescent antibody-stained smears are not recommended for the diagnosis of gonorrhea in women except as an adjunct to the cultures.
   B. Neither the delayed fluorescent antibody-stained smears nor the delayed fluorescent antibody procedure is recommended as a test of cure in women.[9,12]

4. Check for other forms of STD in all patients. For example, all patients with gonorrhea should be examined for coexisting syphilis (which may be concealed by gonorrheal chemotherapy), condylomata acuminata, herpes infection, etc.

Recommended Diagnostic Approach*

1. Vaginal symptoms — Exudate (discharge), pruritus (itching) and/or dyspareunia (painful sexual intercourse).
   A. Gram stain and culture from endocervix and culture pharynx and rectum as a screen for *N. gonorrhoeae*.

---

*From the Pennsylvania Department of Public Health, Division of Acute Infectious Diseases, Harrisburg, Pennsylvania, 1984.

B. Gram stain of exudate.
   (1) *N. gonorrhoeae* — Treat the patient for gonorrhea if the gram stain reveals typical biscuit-shaped gram-negative intracellular diplococci within polymorphonuclear leukocytes.
   (2) *Gardnerella vaginale* — Clue cells or large numbers of typical organisms present requires the definitive treatment for such.
   (3) *Candida* — Treat the patient for candida vaginalis vaginitis if the organism is present in large numbers or if no other pathogens are isolated.
C. Wet Prep — Trichomonas vaginalis vaginitis — Treat the patient if this disease is present. Approximately 50 percent of women with gonococcal cervicitis have this infection as well.[10]
D. If the gram stain and wet prep are negative, a Giemsa stain should be performed looking for trichomonas.
E. If all of the above etiological agents are absent, treat the patient for nonspecific vaginitis.
F. For patients with persistent exudate or post-treatment symptoms:
   (1) Reevaluate the above diagnostic and treatment protocol.
   (2) If the reevaluation does not provide diagnosis, work up the patient's contacts and culture the patient for trichomoniasis, candidiasis, gardnerella vaginale (if possible) and treat whatever infection reveals itself.

2. Abdominal pain, with or without vaginal symptoms:
A. Work up as for **vaginal symptoms**.
B. Consider pelvic inflammatory disease (salpingitis) if there is lower quadrant abdominal pain particularly upon movement, if there is adnexal tenderness, or tenderness upon moving the cervix on bimanual examination.
C. Consider hospital admission if severe PID is present, if abscess is possible, if the diagnosis is uncertain, if the patient is pregnant, if the patient is nauseated or vomiting (and unable to consume oral medications), and in instances where there is failure to respond to therapy.

3. Inguinal lymphadenopathy or adenitis — Either unilateral or bilateral (one or both sides of the groin respectively).
A. Perform a pelvic examination — Check for lesions associated with syphilis, herpes progenitalis, chancroid, condyloma accuminata, etc.
B. Consider the possibility of infection with lymphogranuloma venereum.
C. Consider the possibility of infection with granuloma inguinale.
D. Examine the patient for generalized lymphadenopathy syndrome (GLS) as a clue for potential systemic disease.

Gonococcal Disease

4. Lesions — Check for the following conditions in attempting to determine the precise diagnosis:
  A. *Condylomata accuminata*
  B. *Granuloma inguinale*
  C. *Herpes progenitalis* — Typical lesions allow for a presumptive diagnosis; Pap or Tzanck smears may be helpful in diagnosis; cultures represent the most sensitive and most specific test if the specimen is obtained from an unbroken vesicle.
  D. *Condylomata lata* — Perform a darkfield examination.
  E. *Syphilis* — Perform a Darkfield examination (Ulcerative-type lesion).
  F. *Chancroid* — Ulcerative — Do G.S. and culture.

5. Rectal symptoms — 70 percent of gonococcal proctitis patients are asymptomatic, with pruritus the most commonly presented symptom in addition to bloody discharge, purulent exudate, diarrhea, constipation, abdominal pain, fever, and fatigue as potential signs and symptoms.[7,39]
  A. Perform a gram stain for *N. gonorrhoeae*. If positive, treat for GC infection; if negative, perform cultures for *N. gonorrhoeae*.
  B. If the gonorrhea work-up is negative, rule out syphilis and consider other diseases such as chlamydia, LGV, syphilis, etc.

6. Contacts — Defined as female patients whose sexual partners have been definitively diagnosed with a specific infectious disease.
  A. *Syphilis* — Perform a thorough examination, history, RPR, cultures; and treat for primary syphilis for contact within 90 days.
  B. *Gonorrhea* — Perform a thorough examination, history, RPR, cultures; and treat for uncomplicated gonorrhea for contact within 30 days.
  C. *Nonspecific nongonococcal urethritis* — Perform a thorough examination, history, RPR, cultures; and treat as for NSU.
  D. *Trichomonal vaginalis vaginitis* — Perform a thorough examination, history, RPR, smear, cultures; and treat for trichomonal infection.

The FTA-ABS for syphilis should be utilized when the RPR fails to produce a fairly definitive diagnosis along with clinical symptomology and darkfield examination.[1,10,33]

The Diagnosis of Gonorrhea in Women — Summary

Diagnosis of acute gonorrhea in females is cumbersome; bacteriologic identification may not be obtained through the utilization of the simple gram stain, but is dependent upon cultural evidence. In females, the diagnosis by the gram stain smear is too insensitive, yielding a high

80 The Sexually Transmitted Diseases

percentage of "false" negatives in the presence of known gonococcal infections. This technique may also yield false positive results due to the presence in the female of saprophytic neisseria which on a smear are morphologically indistinguishable from *Neisseria gonorrhoeae*. Culture specimens should be obtained from the endocervical canal, pharynx, and rectal canal. While the cervix is the primary site for gonococcal infections in females, approximately 10 percent of females are positive only for gonococcal proctitis (rectal gonorrhea).[31] Approximately 70 percent of rectal gonorrhea is asymptomatic.[7,10,16,17]

Diagnosis — Laboratory Techniques

Culture Specimen Technique for Men

1. Urethral culture — Indicated when a gram stain of mucopurulent urethral exudate is not positive, in tests of cure, or as test for incubating gonorrhea. Use a cotton swab or sterile bacteriological wire loop and insert in approximately one-half inch into the urethra to obtain specimen from the anterior urethra by gently scraping the mucosal tissues. The diagnostic technique is more painful but no more accurate should the swab or loop be inserted further than one-half inch into the urethra.[10]

2. Anal canal culture — These can be taken with a cotton swab inserted approximately one inch into the rectum, allowing a few seconds for absorption of exudate and utilizing another swab should it come into contact with feces.

3. Pharyngeal culture — Deeply swab the pharynx, including the tonsilar area; examination may reveal pharyngeal erythema, edema, and exudate along with pharyngeal pain and cervical lymphadenopathy. The patient should be examined for a potential peritonsillar abscess, which may ultimately cause apnea if severe in sleeping patients (often on analgesics for pain relief).

Culture Specimen Technique for Women

1. Cervical culture — The cervix is the best site to culture. Moisten the speculum with *warm water*; do not utilize any other lubricant. Remove cervical mucus, preferably with a cotton ball held in ring forceps. Insert a sterile cotton-tipped swab into the endocervical canal; move the swab from side to side, allowing several seconds for absorption of the organisms upon the swab.

2. **Anal canal culture** — This is the site most likely to be positive if there is no gonococcal cervicitis. This specimen can be easily obtained after the cervical specimen without changing the patient's position or utilizing an anoscope. Insert a sterile cotton-tipped swab into the rectal canal approximately one inch; use another swab should the first come into contact with feces. Move the swab from side to side to sample crypts, allowing several seconds for absorption of the organisms upon the swab.

3. **Pharyngeal cultures** — The pharynx should be deeply and carefully swabbed, including the tonsillar region. The patient should be examined for peritonsillar abscess. Owen found that only 3 of 11 patients with gonococcal pharyngitis had symptoms — typical symptoms of other forms of pharyngitis such as erythema, pain, mucus exudate, fever, cervical lymphadenopathy, and fatigue.[10]

4. **Urethral and vaginal cultures** — Indicated when the cervical culture is unsatisfactory as with hysterectomy patients, children, or when maximal sensitivity is desired such as in special medicolegal, social, or research situations.
   - A. *Urethral culture* — Strip the urethra toward the orifice to express an exudate, a process known as "milking" the urethra with digital pressure.[1,10] Utilize a sterile bacteriological wire loop or sterile cotton-tipped swab to obtain the specimen. The wire loop is generally less painful to patients.
   - B. *Vaginal culture* — Utilize a speculum to obtain a specimen from the posterior vaginal vault, or obtain the specimen from the vaginal orifice if the hymen membrane is intact.

Inoculation Upon Thayer-Martin or Transgrow Medium

1. **Thayer-Martin Plates**
   - A. Roll the swab directly upon the Thayer-Martin medium in a large "Z" pattern to provide adequate exposure of the swab to plate for the transfer of organisms. A less desirable alternative is to place the swab in a holding medium and refrigerate it until plating.
   - B. Cross-streak immediately with a sterile wire loop, preferably in the clinic. If not done previously, cross streaking should be done in the laboratory.
   - C. Place the culture in a candle jar as soon as possible.
   - D. Begin incubation of the plates the same day.

Cultural identification of *Neisseria gonorrhoeae*, once a laborious procedure, has been greatly simplified with the advent of Thayer-Martin media. Thayer-Martin media allow the growth of pathogenic *N.*

gonorrhoeae and *N. meningitidis* while greatly inhibiting saprophytic *Neisseria* and other contaminants. This selectivity is especially important in the diagnosis of acute gonorrhea, since specimens must be routinely obtained from heavily contaminated areas such as the cervix and anal canal. If the specimens inoculated upon Thayer-Martin medium demonstrate typical colonial morphology, are positive for gram-stain as gram-negative intracellular diplococci from the colony and demonstrate positive oxidase reaction with one percent dimethyl-p-phenylenediamine hydrochloride, a presumptive diagnosis of gonorrhea can be made with confidence.[31] Special tests such as sugar fermentation or fluorescent antibody are not required unless special circumstances prevail, such as medicolegal situations, where a definitive diagnosis is required. In such instances, sugar fermentation is valuable in differentiating *N. gonorrhoeae* from *N. meningitidis* in those instances where specimens were obtained from blood, spinal, or joint fluid. *N. gonorrhoeae* will ferment only glucose while *N. meningitidis* will ferment both glucose and maltose, thus permitting differentiation. Fluorescent antibody staining for *N. gonorrhoeae* should be reserved as another confirmatory procedure for organisms already isolated on Thayer-Martin media.

All patients with gonorrhea should be carefully examined to rule out syphilis and/or other forms of STD. To detect incubating syphilis or syphilis which might be concealed by gonorrheal chemotherapy, all patients who do not receive the recommended amount of penicillin for therapy should have a serologic test for syphilis performed at the time of treatment and each month thereafter for a total of four months.[31]

2. Transgrow bottles — Inoculate specimens upon the surface of Transgrow medium as follows:

    A. Caution — Keep the neck of the bottle in an elevated position to minimize carbon dioxide loss. Remove the cap of the bottle only when ready to inoculate the medium.

    B. Soak up all excess moisture in the bottle with the specimen swab and then roll the swab from side to side across the medium, starting at the bottom of the bottle.

    C. When feasible, incubate the Transgrow bottle in an upright position at 35–37°C for 16–18 hours before mailing it, noting this on the request form. Resultant growth survives prolonged transport and is ready for identification upon arrival at the laboratory.

    D. Package the capped Transgrow bottle and the request form in an appropriate container to prevent potential breakage, and immediately transport the package to a central bacteriological laboratory by the U.S. Postal Service or by other reliable and convenient means.

    E. At the laboratory, the preincubated Transgrow bottles will be examined immediately for *Neisseria gonorrhoeae*; other bottles will be incubated at 35–37°C for 24–48 hours and examined.[9]

Transgrow, a selective medium for the transport and cultivation of *N. gonorrhoeae*, is utilized for sending specimens to a central laboratory; Thayer-Martin (TM) plates are utilized when there is an immediate access to a laboratory.[42] Transgrow medium under ten percent carbon dioxide atmosphere in bottles promotes growth of pathogenic *Neisseria* and suppresses contaminating organisms similarly to Thayer-Martin medium in plates. Transgrow medium maintains viability of pathogenic *Neisseria* for more than 48 hours at room temperature. Validity of culture results depends upon proper techniques for obtaining, inoculating, and the handling of specimens.[9,42]

Preliminary evaluation indicates that the storage or shelf-life of Transgrow medium at room temperature may be in excess of three months. Many physicians and laboratories are utilizing Transgrow medium; however, unsatisfactory results are possible unless physicians practice proper techniques in obtaining and inoculating specimens and unless microbiologists become more familiar with appropriate procedures and follow them carefully.[9,42] Colonial morphology may be atypical on Transgrow medium.[9,42]

Laboratory Techniques for the Diagnosis of Gonorrhea Under Special Circumstances*

In special, social, medicolegal, and research situations when specific identification of organisms isolated upon either Thayer-Martin (TM) or Transgrow medium from the pharyngeal or anogenital region is desired, fermentation reactions should be utilized to confirm an identification of *Neisseria gonorrhoeae*. Fluorescent antibody staining can be utilized as a confirmatory test for organisms isolated on either medium if insufficient isolated colonies of suspected gonococci are available for inoculation of fermentation medium or if the organisms are no longer viable.[9,42]

Culture on TM medium is the diagnostic procedure of choice in special situations such as suspected gonococcal conjunctivitis, gonococcal arthritis, gonococcal septicemia, etc. Identification of *N. gonorrhoeae* should be confirmed as described in item one above.

Gram staining and fluorescent antibody staining of smears from conjunctivae, joint fluids, or skin lesions can be utilized as an adjunct in the diagnosis of these manifestations of gonorrhea, particularly when partial therapy may prevent cultural recovery of organisms. (Fluorescent antibody conjugates are check-tested for specificity by the sexually transmitted disease (STD) laboratory for utilization only in a confirmatory test for

---

*From the Communicable Disease Center, Atlanta, Georgia.

organisms grown on selective media, and not for staining of direct smears).[9,42]

Specific Diagnosis and Recommended Chemotherapy for Uncomplicated Gonorrhea*

Gonococcal Urethritis

1. Major Symptomology — Mucopurulent urethral exudate; dysuria; frequency; inguinal lymphadenopathy; fever.

2. Diagnosis — Gram stain microscopic identification of gram-negative intracellular diplococci in a smear of urethral exudate; cultures of the urethra and other potentially infected orifices (pharynx, rectum, cervix).

3. Treatment — Tetracycline HCL 500 mg p.o.,q.i.d. for 7 days (total of 14 gms) *or* Penicillin G. procaine 4.8 million units (MU) I.M. in 2 sites plus 1 gm probenecid p.o. (orally) just prior to the injection; Ampicillin 3.5 gm p.o. plus 1 gm of probenecid.

4. Alternative Treatment — Spectinomycin 2 gm I.M.; Cefoxitin 2 gm I.M. plus 1.0 gm probenecid, and Cefotaxime 1.0 gm I.M. are all utilized for penicillin-resistant gonorrhea.

Gonococcal Cervicitis

1. Major Symptomology — Approximately 75 to 90 percent of women are asymptomatic; those with symptomology present with a potential exudate and dysuria.[1,10,16,17]

2. Diagnosis — Gram stain of exudate and/or culture of the endocervix.

3. Treatment — see *Gonococcal Urethritis*.

4. Alternative Treatment — The same as for gonococcal urethritis; however, tetracycline hydrochloride must *not* be given to pregnant women

---

*From the Pennsylvania Department of Public Health, Division of Infectious Diseases, and the Communicable Disease Center of Atlanta, Georgia, unless otherwise noted.

as it could cause fetal death due to liver damage, bone destruction and mottled (stained) primary and secondary teeth.[1,10] Penicillin and ampicillin can be given to nonallergic pregnant women; erythromycin and spectinomycin have also been utilized.[10] Natural penicillin G is destroyed by stomach acid and therefore cannot be given orally (p.o.); ampicillin is a semisynthetic form of penicillin which is not destroyed by stomach acid. Ampicillin with 1 gm of probenecid is 93 percent effective in producing definitive therapy; approximately five percent of Americans are allergic to penicillin, which could produce potentially fatal anaphylactoid or anaphylactic shock. Tetracycline injected is extremely painful; thus it should be given orally upon an empty stomach as its absorption is reduced by food. Eating should be delayed for at least one hour.[10] Side effects of tetracycline include digestive irritation, nausea, vomiting, diarrhea, abnormal skin sensitivity to sunlight, and intestinal suprainfections.[10] Intestinal suprainfections are rare but potentially fatal if not promptly treated; symptomology includes fever and severe diarrhea, with liquid feces containing blood or shreds of membranes from the intestinal walls.[10]

Pelvic Inflammatory Disease (Gonococcal Salpingitis)*

1. Major Symptomology — Abdominal pain bilaterally generally in the lower quadrants; a longer and more painful menstrual period; nausea and vomiting; hyperpyrexia over 102°F; pain during sexual intercourse; abnormal vaginal bleeding; with subacute salpingitis difficult to diagnose. There may be abdominal pain on moving and tenderness during the pelvic examination in the adnexal regions when the cervix is moved.[1,10,39]

2. Diagnosis — Clinical presentation, gram stain, and cultures.

3. Treatment — Outpatient: Tetracycline HCL 500 mg p.o., q.i.d. for 10 days *or*: Penicillin G procaine 4.8 MU/IM in 2 sites plus 1 gm of probenecid p.o., just prior to the injection followed by Tetracycline HCL 500 mg p.o., q.i.d. for 10 days. (Ampicillin 3.5 gm p.o. or Amoxicillin 3.0 gm p.o. may be utilized instead of Penicillin G procaine). Inpatient: Cefoxitin 2 gm IV q.i.d. for 10 days. If chlamydia is suspected, add tetracycline

---

*This treatment regimen assumes a *gonococcal etiology*; it must be emphasized that not all PID is gonococcal and that other organisms (*Bacteroides fragilis*, gram-negative enterics, and chlamydiae) may warrant consideration as well based upon the patient's clinical response and cervical and cul-de-sac cultures and smear.

HCL 250 IV q.i.d. until the patient shows improvement, then give 500 mg p.o., q.i.d. for 10 days.*

4. Alternative Treatment — Outpatient: Cefoxitin 2gm IM plus 1 gm probenecid p.o. plus tetracycline HCL 500 mg p.o., q.i.d. for 10 days. Inpatient: Several other agents are available, depending upon the likelihood of the presence of anerobes (Clindamycin) or gram-negative enteric bacilli (Gentamicin).

Gonococcal Proctitis

1. Major Symptomology — Approximately 70 percent of patients with gonococcal proctitis are asymptomatic.[7,10,16,17] The most common symptoms include: Itching, bloody and/or mucous discharge, rectal pain, diarrhea, constipation, a sense of incomplete evacuation of the bowel, abdominal pain, and fever.[1,10,39]

2. Diagnosis — Gram stain culture, the effectiveness of which is questioned by some medical authorities in terms of definitive diagnosis.[37,43]

3. Treatment — Penicillin G. procaine 4.8 MU/IM in 2 sites plus 1 Gm probenecid p.o. just prior to the injection.

4. Alternative Treatment — Spectinomycin 2 Gm IM; Cefoxitin 2 GM IM plus 1.0 Gm probenecid; Cefotaxime 1.0 Gm IM. All are useful for penicillin-resistant gonococci.

Gonococcal Pharyngitis

1. Major Symptomology — Approximately 70 percent of patients with gonococcal pharyngitis are asymptomatic; those with symptoms present symptoms for other forms of pharyngitis: Erythema, exudate, pain, tonsillitis, cervical lymphadenopathy, and potential fever.

2. Diagnosis — Gram stain and cultures.

3. Treatment — Tetracycline HCL 500 m.g. p.o. q.i.d. for 7 days (14 gm total) *or* Penicillin G procaine 4.8 MU/IM in 2 sites plus 1 gm pro-

---

*The patient should be hospitalized if the diagnosis is idiopathic, if abscess is possible, if pregnant, if nauseated and vomiting, and if there is failure to respond to therapy. Follow-up for response to treatment in the first 24–48 hours is strongly advised.

benecid p.o. just prior to the injection. Tetracycline is not to be utilized for children under 8 years of age or for pregnant patients. It may be absorbed poorly if taken with food and dairy products, and it is less preferable than a single-dose regimen in patients who are unlikely to complete a multiple dose regimen.

4. Alternative Treatment — Neither Spectinomycin nor a single dose of Ampicillin is currently recommended. For resistance, Sulfamethoxazole trimethoprim 9 tablets (400 mg sulfamethoxazole/80 mg trimethoprim per tablet) daily for 5 days.

Specific Diagnosis and Recommended Treatment for Complicated Gonorrhea

Metastatic Gonorrhea or Disseminated Gonococcal Infection (DGI)

1. Major Symptomology — Gonococcal septicemia; 50 percent of patients develop gonococcal dermatitis, arthralgia, fever, and arthritis.

2. Diagnosis — Culture of blood, skin lesions, urethra, cervix, rectum, and pharynx, gram stain of skin lesions, urethral or cervical exudate.

3. Treatment — Penicillin G Crystalline 10 MU/IV daily until there is improvement followed by Ampicillin 500 mg q.i.d. for 7 days of therapy.

4. Alternative Treatment — Ampicillin 3.5 gm p.o., plus probenecid 1 gm followed by Ampicillin 500 mg p.o., q.i.d. for 7 days. Tetracycline HCL or erythromycin p.o., q.i.d. for 7 days (for a total of 14 gms) may be given. Cefoxitin 1.0 gm or Cefotaxime 5 gms q.i.d. IV for 5 days (treatment of choice for DGI caused by PPNG).

Gonococcal Infection During Pregnancy

Same as for gonococcal cervicitis, except do *not* prescribe tetracycline HCL as it can cause death of the fetus from liver damage as well as bone destruction and mottling of the infant's primary and secondary teeth.[1,10] Penicillin, ampicillin, erythromycin, and spectinomycin may be utilized with pregnant women.

Gonococcal Meningitis

1. **Major Symptomology** — Fever, stiff neck, and headache.

2. **Diagnosis** — Refer for hospitalization; smear and culture of the spinal fluid.

3. **Treatment** — Penicillin G Crystalline, 12-24 MU/IV daily for at least 10 days.

4. **Alternative Treatment** — Chloramphenicol 1.0 gm IV every 6 hours for at least 10 days or Moxalactam 2.0 gm IV every 6 hours for at least 10 days.

Gonococcal Endocarditis

1. **Major Symptomology** — Fever, murmur, petechiae (hemorrhagic rash), and hematuria (blood in the urine).

2. **Diagnosis** — Refer for hospitalization; blood cultures.

3. **Treatment** — Penicillin G Crystaline, 12-24 MU/IV daily for 4 weeks.

4. **Alternative Treatment** — Cefoxitin 2.0 gm or Cefotaxime 1.0 gm IV q.i.d. for 4 weeks.

Gonococcal Adult Ophthalmia or Gonococcal Adult Conjunctivitis

1. **Major Symptoms** — Acute severe conjunctivitis.

2. **Diagnosis** — Refer for hospitalization; smear and culture of exudate.

3. **Treatment** — Penicillin G Crystalline, 10 MU/IV daily for 5 days.

4. **Alternative Treatment** — Cefoxitin 1.0 gm or Cefotaxime .5 gm IV q.i.d. for 5 days.

The Treatment of Gonorrhea in Children*

Infant Born to Mother with Gonorrhea

   1. **Major Symptoms** – None.

   2. **Diagnosis** – Culture and treat immediately.

   3. **Treatment** – Aqueous Crystalline Penicillin G 50,000 U to full-term infants or 20,000 to low birthweight infants, in a single IM injection or IV. The mother and her contact(s) should be completely cultured and treated immediately.

   4. **Alternative Treatment** – Consultation is strongly recommended.

Gonococcal Ophthalmia in Children (Highly Contagious)

   1. **Major Symptoms** – Profuse and purulent exudate, erythema, and edema.

   2. **Diagnosis** – Gram stain, complete cultures.

   3. **Treatment** – Aqueous Crystalline Penicillin G 50,000 U per kg per day IV in 2 dosages for 7 days, along with saline irrigation of the eyes. In older children, increasing the dosage to 100,000 U per kg per day IV is indicated. The mother and her contact(s) should be completely cultured and treated immediately for GC infection and other potential forms of STD.

   4. **Alternative Treatment** – Consultation is strongly recommended.

Gonococcal Vulvovaginitis, Urethritis, Proctitis, and/or Pharyngitis in Children

   1. **Major Symptomology** – Same as for gonococcal disease in adults.

   2. **Diagnosis** – Gram stain and complete cultures.

---

*Children weighing more than 100 lbs (45 kilograms) should be treated with adult dosages.[34]

3. **Treatment** — Aqueous Procaine Penicillin G 100,000 U per kg IM plus probenecid 25 mg per kg (maximum of 1 gm) or Amoxicillin 50 mg per kg p.o. with probenecid 25 mg per kg (maximum of 1 gm).*

Pediatric Metastatic Gonorrhea or Pediatric Disseminated Gonococcal Infection (DGI)

1. **Major Symptomology** — Same as for gonococcal disease in adults.

2. **Diagnosis** — Cultures of blood, etc., same as for adult DGI.

3. **Treatment** — Aqueous Crystalline Penicillin G — 100,000 per kg per day IV in two or three divided doses for 7 days. Meningitis in the neonate should be treated with Aqueous Crystalline Penicillin G — 100,000 U per kg per day IV divided into three or four dosages and continued for 10 days. In older children, meningitis should be treated with Aqueous Crystalline Penicillin G — 250,000 U per kg per day IV in six divided dosages for at least 10 days.

4. **Alternative Treatment** — With the exception of tetracycline HCL in children under 8 years of age for treatment of complicated disease, the alternative regimens recommended for adults may be utilized in appropriate pediatric dosages.[39]

Pennsylvania Act 124 defines child abuse as serious physical or mental injury unexplained by past history as being accidental, or sexual abuse, or serious physical neglect, when that harm is caused by "acts or omissions" of the parents or guardians. All health personnel are required to report suspected child abuse in all 50 states; to report suspected child abuse, call "Childline" at 1-800-932-0313.

Penicillinase-Producing Neisseria Gonorrhoeae (PPNG)*

A strain of gonococci resistant to all forms of penicillin emerged early in 1976 with implications for the treatment, control, and eventual eradication of gonorrhea. In 1976, evidence of PPNG was first noted on American military bases and adjacent cities in the Republic of the Philippines. Since then, these strains have been reported by 18 countries, including Australia,

---

*From the Center for Disease Control, Atlanta, Georgia, and the U.S. Public Health Service.

Belgium, Canada, Denmark, England, Ghana, Hong Kong, Japan, the Netherlands, New Zealand, Norway, the Philippines, Republic of Korea, Singapore, South Africa, Sweden, Switzerland, and the United States.

From March 1976 through December 1977, 288 cases of PPNG were identified in 28 States and Guam. The results of the interview contact-referral procedure applied to PPNG cases detected in the United States demonstrated that a significant proportion was related to importation of the infection from either southeast Asia or the west coast of Africa. Surveillance efforts include the testing of patients after treatment by culturing for the presence of PPNG and, in selected regions, screening all cultures. Control measures have included intensive field investigations and the referral of sexual partners for epidemiological treatment.

The Medical Treatment for Suspected or Proven Cases of Penicillin Resistance*

1. Gonococcal Urethritis, Proctitis, and/or Cervicitis — Spectinomycin 2 gm/IM. For treatment failures — Cefoxitin 2 gm/IM plus 1.0 gm probenecid, *or* Cefoxamine 1.0 gm IM.

2. Gonococcal Pharyngitis — Sulfamethoxazole — Trimethoprim 9 tablets (400 mg sulfamethoxazole/80 mg trimethoprim per tablet) daily for 5 days.

3. Gonococcal Pelvic Inflammatory Disease (PID) — Outpatient: Spectinomycin 2 gm/IM daily for 5 to 10 days. Inpatient: Cefoxitin 2 gm/IV every 6 hours for 10 days.

4. Metastatic Gonorrhea — Disseminated Gonococcal Infection — Cefoxitin 1.0 gm *or* Cefotaxime .5 gm q.i.d. IV for 5 days.

5. Adult Gonococcal Conjunctivitis — Cefoxitin 1.0 gm *or* Cefotaxime .5 gm 4 times daily IV for 5 days.

Note: Spectinomycin 2 gm IM is now recommended for the initial treatment of uncomplicated gonococcal proctitis in patients who have recently returned from countries such as the Phillipines, Singapore, and Thailand — areas of high prevalence of PPNG infections.[39] All gonorrhea patients should have a test-for-cure within one week of chemotherapy; all positive test-of-cures should be tested for penicillin sensitivity and betalactamase.[39]

---

*From the Pennsylvania Department of Public Health, Division of Acute Infectious Diseases.

Response and Retreatment

Patient Response to Chemotherapy

More than 90 percent of gonococcal infections are definitively treated with prompt penicillin treatment.[44] Tetracycline, erythromycin, and other antibiotics may be effectively utilized for patients allergic to penicillin.[44] The exudate disappears generally within 12 hours as most of the gonococci are killed within two to nine hours.[10,44] A thin flow of exudate may persist for a few days in approximately 10-15 percent of patients.[10,44] The patient is generally noncontagious within 24 hours following chemotherapy, particularly with penicillin and ampicillin injected or taken orally in massive dosages. All symptomology may disappear within two to three days; the patient is encouraged to avoid sexual contact for approximately five days.

Post-Treatment Evaluation

All patients with gonorrhea should receive posttreatment evaluation one week following treatment. Tests-of-cure are mandatory in the proper management of gonorrhea patients—particularly women and homosexual or bisexual males.[1,10,16,17] The urethra, pharynx, cervix, vagina, and rectum should be carefully cultured if any possibility for infection exists; all gonorrhea patients should receive an RPR and an FTA-ABS in instances where such is indicated. All patients should be given careful consideration for other forms of STD.[1,10,16,17,31] As asymptomology following treatment is often believed to constitute cure, often tests-of-cure are omitted.[1,10,31]

Gonorrhea patients who fail to respond to initial chemotherapy and who are without evidence of reinfection should be retreated according to the following schedule:[31]

1. Females.—4.8 million units of aqueous procaine penicillin G (APPG) IM on 2 successive days for a total of *9.6 million units of APPG.*

2. Males.—4.8 million units of aqueous procaine penicillin G (APPG) IM at one visit; gay and bisexual males with gonococcal proctitis should be given the dosage for females, in the opinion of many medical authorities.[1,9,10,35] Thus, the treatment of complications of gonorrhea must be individualized, utilizing large amounts of short-acting penicillin (aqueous procaine penicillin G).[31]

Chemotherapeutic Precautions and Contradictions for Gonococcal Disease

1. Neither Penicillin G. Benzathine (most often supplied as Bicillin) nor oral penicillin G has any place in the treatment of gonorrhea.[39]

2. Tetracycline HCL.—Must *not* be given to pregnant women, as liver damage fatal to the fetus, bone destruction, and mottling of the infant's primary and secondary teeth may result. Caution must be exercised in regard to sun exposure, as this drug increases one's sensitivity to sunlight.[10] The drug may be absorbed poorly if taken with food, dairy products, and iron.[10,39] Tetracycline injected is extremely painful; thus it is always given orally with food intake delayed preferably for at least 2 hours. Tetracycline hydrochloride should *not* be utilized for children under 8 years of age;[39] it is generally less preferable than a single dosage regimen for patients unlikely to complete a multi-dosage regimen.[39]

Some of the major side effects of tetracycline HCL internalization include digestive irritation (heartburn), nausea, vomiting, diarrhea, abnormal skin sensitivity to sunlight, anaphylactoid and anaphylactic shock, transient arthritis on large ingestions, and rare suprainfections of the intestine in which normal bacteria helpful to digestion are destroyed which prevent the growth of pathogenic organisms.[10] In most instances, these helpful bacteria repopulate within the intestines a few days following the end of tetracycline chemotherapy. Approximately five percent of patients develop the suprainfection, characterized by fever, severe diarrhea, blood within liquid feces, and death without adequate prompt treatment.[1,10,33]

An unknown percentage of the U.S. population is allergic to penicillin. Both anaphylactoid (first exposure) and anaphylactic (subsequent exposure) shock may arise from internalization of tetracycline hydrochloride. Potential signs and symptoms of these forms of shock include weak and rapid pulse (over 100/minute); systolic hypotension (under 100 mg/hg); headache; edema of the lips, tongue, face, etc.; abdominal pain and/or backache; sudden collapse; loss of bowel and bladder control; vertigo; dyspnea (breathing difficulty); angioneurotic edema of the airway (swelling leading to potential airway obstruction); erythema of the skin (flushing); pruritus of the skin (itching); history of previous allergic response; history of prescribed medication; history of allergy to shellfish or strawberry ingestion in particular; burning eyes; skin rash (uticaria—hives); and weakness.[1,10,33]

3. Probenecid.—Taken orally with ampicillin and with injected penicillin, it potentiates the action of the penicillin.[10,33] Probenecid utilization with patients with G-6/PD deficiency may cause hemolytic anemia. While this condition is more common in black males (13 percent), it affects caucasian males (.7 percent) as well.[10] Side effects of probenecid include nausea and vomiting; hypersensitivity; the neprotic syndrome; hepatic injury; and rarely, aplastic anemia.[1,10] Probenecid utilization with patients who excrete excessive quantities of uric acid or who drink little fluid may develop uric acid stones.[1,10,33] Probenecid utilization may precipitate acute gout in susceptible patients.[1,10,33]

4. **Pediatric.**—Children weighing more than 100 lbs (45 kilograms) should be treated with adult dosages.[39]

Contraindicated Chemotherapy for Gonococcal Infections

The following drugs should not be utilized as chemotherapeutic agents for gonorrhea treatment:[10,42] *Streptomycin* and *Kanamycin*, which produce serious side effects, including deafness and renal damage; *Chloramphenicol*, which may cause an acutely fatal aplastic anemia; and *Hetacillin*, a useless "me-too" drug coverted by the human organism into ampicillin without any added therapeutic advantage.

The "ideal" chemotherapeutic agents for gonorrhea would possess the following qualitative characteristics:

- Highly effective in killing gonococci.
- Free of toxic or side effects.
- Economical for all concerned.
- Taken orally in one dose.
- Provide high medication-tissue concentrations.
- Absorption and blood levels could be easily predicted.

Major Causes of Gonorrhea Treatment Failure

1. **Patient Factors:**
   A. Reinfection.
   B. Failure of the patient to return within one week for a test-of-cure.
   C. Failure to abstain from sexual relations for approximately five or more days.
   D. Failure to take the medication properly as prescribed.

2. **Site of Infection:**
   A. Closed focus provides for difficult diagnosis as with gonococcal cervicitis in women and as with gonococcal pharyngitis and gonococcal proctitis.
   B. Incorrect initial diagnosis.
   C. Mixed infection initially.

3. Pharmacological Factors:
   A. Poor absorption.
   B. Drug interaction.
   C. Incorrect drug or formulation.
   D. Too low or too short blood levels.
   E. Antibiotic-insensitive organism.

7. Granuloma Inguinale

Granuloma inguinale (also donovaniasis or granuloma venereum) is a chronic, progressive, ulcerative, autoinoculable, and granulomatous disease generally confined to the skin and mucous mmembranes of the genitoinguinal region but occasionally appearing upon other portions of the body.[1,6,33] The disease is mildly communicable and is nonfatal in nature, with sporadic occurrence within the United States.[1,6,33] As this disease is relatively rare, its precise nature is not understood in many respects.[6]

Occurrence

Granuloma inguinale is an infrequent disease of tropical, subtropical, and temperate regions. It is apparently more common among males than females, and apparently more common among individuals constituting the lower socioeconomic status groups.[6] The disease predominantly affects those within the age group of 20 to 40 years and is seen most among those commonly affected by other forms of sexually transmitted diseases.[1,10,17,33] While the disease is particularly common to the tropics, it has been found to exist in almost every country and climate; the majority of cases within the United States are in the southeastern section, mainly affecting blacks.[33] Only 73 cases of the disease were reported in 1973, in comparison to 165 cases in 1966. The incidence and prevalence of this disease have decreased significantly within the past decade.[33]

Infectious Agent

The etiological agent of granuloma inguinale is a nonmotile, gram-negative bacillus known as the Donovan body (*Donovania granulomatis*).[1,6,8,17] In stained smears of the lesions, the organisms appear as encapsulated, bipolar bodies situated within large mononuclear cells. In chick embryo cultures, the morphology of the organism is variable and may consist of bipolar forms, curved rods, chains, or unencapsulated bodies.[33] The organism is not pathogenic for laboratory animals and can be cultivated only within artificial media containing yolk material.[8,33]

Reservoir and Source of Infection

The reservoir is mankind; the source of infection is probably the active lesions of infected persons.[6,52]

Mode of Transmission

The mode of transmission is idiopathic (unknown); veneral transmission is presumably the principal means of spread, although the disease is not always communicated to regular sexual partners of those infected.[6,33] The Communicable Disease Center notes that spread by autoinoculation is common.[12]

Incubation Period

The incubation period for granuloma inguinale can vary from 8 days to 12 weeks.[1,6,17]

Period of Communicability

Communicability is idiopathic, but presumably most likely while open lesions exist upon the skin or mucous membranes.[1,6,10,33,52]

Susceptibility and Resistance

The susceptibility for this disease is variable; immunity apparently does not follow an attack of disease.[6] The disease is not highly infectious as it is not always contracted by the regular sexual partners of those infected.[1,6,10,33] The factors predisposing to invasion of the organism are not clearly understood; however, the disease is seen most among those commonly contracting other forms of sexually transmitted diseases.[33] In debilitated and neglected cases the ulcerations spread, covering the entire pudendal region, lower abdomen, buttocks, and thighs; these patients commonly become anemic, bedridden, cachectic, and die.[1]

Signs and Symptoms

1. Lesions. — Within 8 days to 12 weeks, a painless vesicle, papule, or nodule appears which may have a beefy-red granular base. The lesions may appear as buttonlike elevations or a granular film covering the glans, with occasional nodules gently bulging the surface.[1] Lesions soon become open lesions, which bleed easily and have a raised, rounded, and velvet-like appearance.[10] The disease is extremely chronic; ulcers slowly enlarge and coalesce, with secondary infections frequent.[33] Lesions about the perineal region closely resemble condylomata lata of secondary syphilis, and darkfield examinations and serologic tests for syphilis should be performed to make a differential diagnosis.[46,52]

   2. **Genital elephantiasis** may occur in instances where there is interference with lymphatic drainage.[33]

   3. **Regional lymphadenopathy.** — Inguinal lymphadenopathy is common in instances of granuloma inguinale.

   4. **Extragenital lesions** have a predilection for warm and moist surfaces such as the folds of the scrotum and thighs or the labia and vagina; if neglected, the disease may result in serious destruction of the genital organs.[1,6,8,10,33]

   5. **Medical history.** — The presence of this disease in one's sexual partner or the presence of other forms of sexually transmitted disease in the patient adds further possible evidence for a diagnosis of this disease

Presumptive Diagnosis*

The typical clinical presentation is sufficient to suggest the presumptive diagnosis. Resolution of the lesions following specific antibiotic therapy supports the diagnosis. A history of travel to the tropics (particularly India or Papua New Guinea) among patients or their sexual partners helps to substantiate the clinical impression.[12]

Definitive Diagnosis*

Scrapings or biopsy specimens from the ulcer margin reveal the pathognomonic Donovan bodies upon microscopic examination. A tissue culture of *C. granulomatis* is not feasible.[12]

Treatment

   1. **Tetracycline.** — .5 gm p.o./q.i.d. for 21 days or until the lesion completely heals; *or*
   2. **Streptomycin.** — .5 gm IM/b.i.d. for at least 21 days; *or*
   3. **Chloramphenicol.** — .5 gm p.o./t.i.d. for at least 21 days; *or*
   4. **Gentamicin.** — 40 mg IM/b.i.d. for at least 21 days.

---

*From the Communicable Disease Center in Atlanta, Georgia.

Erythromycin and sulfamethoxazole/trimethoprim regimens have also been reported to be effective; *penicillins are not effective.*[12]

The patient should return for evaluation 3 to 5 days after the initial visit. Sexual partners should be examined and treated as necessary. The patient should return to the physician weekly or biweekly for evaluation until the infection is entirely healed.[12]

8. Group B Hemolytic Streptococcal Infections

Aerobic streptococci as a group are among the most important bacterial pathogens of mankind; they can invade any body organ or tissue and, depending upon the site of invasion and the parasite-host relationship, produce different clinical syndromes.[33] Streptococcal infections can be divided into two large groups: (1) the acute and often dramatic illnesses, such as streptococcal pharyngitis, scarlet fever, erysipelas, puerperal fever, and lymphangitis, which occur frequently and are characterized by certain toxic, septic, or suppurative features; and (2) the late, nonsuppurative complications of streptococcal infections, including acute glomerulonephritis and acute rheumatic fever, which commonly become manifest 2 and 3 weeks respectively following an acute streptococcal infection.[1,8,33]

Streptococcal infections may also be classified microbially according to the characteristics of the streptococcus, and clinically according to the type of infection.[1] Streptococci are gram-positive bacteria which tend to form in chains and which can be divided into 3 major groups when grown upon sheep blood agar.[1,33] *Alpha colonies* show a zone of incomplete or green hemolysis; *beta colonies* exhibit a clear zone of complete hemolysis; and *gamma colonies* produce no hemolysis.[1,33] Streaking a culture upon a blood agar plate is sufficient to indicate important pathogenic streptococci, as those exhibiting beta hemolysis are responsible for the majority of human infections.[33]

An additional classification, based upon the carbohydrates present within the cell wall, divides streptococci into *Lancefield groups A to O*.[1,33] *Group A hemolytic streptococci* comprise at least 40 specific types, determined by either an agglutinin reaction based upon the T-substance or by the precipitin test, for which the M-substance is the type-specific antigen. Group A streptococci, represented by S-pyogenes, cause a wide variety of diseases clinically differentiated by the portal of entry, tissue locatization of the infectious agent, and the presence or absence of a scarlatinal rash.[6] The most important conditions caused by Group A streptococci are scarlet fever, streptococcal pharyngitis, erysipelas, puerperal fever, cellulitis, lymphadenitis, septicemia, impetigo contagiosa, and other forms of skin and wound infections.[6] *Group B Streptococci* may cause sexually transmitted disease along with neonatal sepsis and meningitis, puerperal infections, urinary tract infections, and endocarditis.[71] *Group C streptococci* may cause skin and wound infections, bacteremias, endocarditis, pharyngitis, with respiratory infections rare.[33,71] Infections due to *group D streptococci enterococci* include endocarditis, peritonitis, and wound and urinary tract infections, while *group D streptococci nonenterococci* cause urinary tract infections along with bacteremia and endocarditis.[71] Infections caused by *group G streptococci* are similar to those of group C, while *groups F, H, and K streptococci* cause sinusitis, meningitis, brain abscesses, pneumonia, and endocarditis.[71] *Nongroupable streptococci* may cause endocarditis, and *anaerobic streptococci* may cause sinusitis, pneumonia, lung abscesses, empyema, brain abscesses, soft tissue infections, and bone and joint infections.[71]

Group B hemolytic streptococci were first recognized as animal pathogens causing bovine mastitis, but are now clearly established as very important pathogens for human infections and now constitute a form of sexually transmitted disease.[27,71] In addition, group B streptococci may cause a broad range of infections in adults.[71]

Occurrence

Group B streptococcal infections are worldwide and can affect all ages and races. Group B streptococcal infections in adults are common, and in one study, these organisms accounted for 2 percent of all neonatal bacteremias and 8 percent of nonneonatal streptococcal bacteremias.[72] The disease is apt to be more common among individuals with a variety of sexual partners; high rates of carriage of group B streptococci were found among men (38 percent) and women (42.3 percent) attending a clinic for sexually transmitted diseases.[72]

Infectious Etiological Agent

Most group B streptococci are beta hemolytic in nature, with 6 to 20 percent sensitive to low-dose bacitracin.[71] Group B streptococci can be presumptively separated from group A streptococci upon the basis of their ability to hydrolyze sodium hippurate; however, definitive identification depends upon immunological identification of the group B carbohydrate.[71] Group B streptococci can be divided into 5 subtypes — Ia, Ib, Ic, II, and III with classification based upon surface polysaccharide and protein antigens.[71]

Reservoir and Source of Infection

The reservoir of infection is mankind; the source of infection is infected saliva, seminal fluid, urine, feces, or vaginal secretions. Streptococcal infections may also arise from respiratory discharges (mainly group A) and occasionally from contaminated food.[33]

Mode of Transmission

Current knowledge suggests that these organisms, as they are contained in some body fluids, may be communicated during sexual activity. An important cause of neonatal sepsis, B hemolytic streptococci may reside within the maternal vagina and infect neonates during passage through the vaginal canal or may be acquired within neonatal nurseries.[72]

Incubation Period

The incubation period for group B hemolytic streptococcal infections is similar to that for other forms of streptococcal infection: generally 1 to 3 days, rarely longer.[6] Two broad syndromes of maternal infection, early onset and late onset, have been reported.[71] Early-onset infection occurs within the first 10 days of life and is associated with prematurity and prolonged rupture of the membranes but can occur after uncomplicated term deliveries and is fulminating. The late-onset syndrome (beyond 10 days of life) is unrelated to obstetric complications, is more insidious in onset, and is often dominated by meningitis.[71]

Period of Communicability

The disease is communicable while the infectious agent resides within saliva, urine, seminal fluid, vaginal secretions, and/or feces.

Susceptibility and Resistance

Susceptibility to this disease appears general, with those engaged in frequent sexual activity with a wide variety of different sexual partners constituting a population at risk. Group B streptococci can cause neonatal infections during birth as well as a wide range of infections in adults. Most patients are women of childbearing age, who often have infection related to parturition or gynecological problems, or elderly patients of either sex, who often have genitourinary disorders, diabetes mellitus, or other debilitating conditions.[71]

Signs and Symptoms — Neonatal Infections

Two broad syndromes, early and late onset, have been noted:

1. **Early onset** occurs within the first 10 days of life and is associated

with prematurity, prolonged rupture of membranes, and a fulminating course of disease. This can also arise following uncomplicated deliveries.[71] Bacteremia and shock are present in most patients, with pneumonia, meningitis, or both seen in 30 to 50 percent of patients; *mortality exceeds 50 percent despite treatment.*[71]

2. Late onset occurs beyond 10 days of life, is unrelated to obstetrical complications, is more insidious in onset and more often dominated by meningitis, with a devastating process but better prognosis (mortality below 30 percent).[71]

Signs and Symptoms — Adult Infections

Group B streptococci can cause a wide range of infections in adults, including bacteremia, endometritis, pyelonephritis, endocarditis, meningitis, pulmonary infections, and infections of skin, soft tissues, and wounds.[71]

Diagnosis

The diagnosis is made by medical history in conjunction with clinical manifestations of disease and laboratory techniques. Swab cultures reveal the presence of the organism; swabs of the anorectal/perineal regions and subpreputial sac have been shown to provide the highest isolation rates, while swab cultures of the urethra have been found to provide the lowest isolation rates.[71] Serotyping and phagetyping may be utilized to reveal the particular strain of the organism involved.[72]

Treatment

1. Penicillin. — Although group B streptococci are sensitive to clinically achievable levels of penicillin, the minimum inhibitory concentrations (MIC) are somewhat higher than those for group A streptococci.[71]

2. Alternative Treatments. — The great majority of group B streptococci are sensitive to cephalosporins, erythromycin, clindamycin, and chloramphenicol but are resistant to tetracycline and kanamycin. Penicillin-gentamicin synergism can be shown in some strains, despite aminoglycoside resistance, but its clinical significance is unknown.[71]

9. Herpes Progenitalis

Herpes represents the family name for approximately 50 related viruses, including herpes virus hominis type 1 and 2 infections along with the virus responsible for infectious mononucleosis (Epstein-Barr virus), chicken pox (varicella), and shingles (herpes zoster).

With respect to sexually transmitted diseases, herpes is the common term for two viral infections presently existing at epidemic proportions within the United States, perhaps affecting as many as 30 million Americans.[16] Herpes simplex virus hominis type 1 (HSV-1) infection generally refers to "cold sores," "fever blisters," or infection above the beltline, while herpes simplex virus hominis type 2 (HSV-2) infection generally refers to genital herpes.[1,10,16,54,55] However, HSV-1 and HSV-2 infections are clinically indistinguishable; their occurrence can be conclusively determined virologically only with a culture.[57]

History

The first known cases of herpes date back to the days of the Roman empire, when for a time it was so prevalent that a ban was placed on kissing.[58] The herpes simplex virus was not isolated until 1912.

Occurrence

It was not until 1965 that herpes infections received considerable attention as a major form of STD; since that time they have increased dramatically, so that herpes presently ranks second only to gonorrhea in venereal incidence and accounts for approximately 13 percent of all sexually transmitted disease within the United States.[16] Studies in various clinics suggest that approximately one case of herpes is diagnosed for every ten cases of gonorrhea.[59] Herpes infections have an estimated prevalence within the U.S. alone of between 20 and 30 million cases, with an estimated 300,000 to 600,000 new cases occurring each year.[16,57,58]

Unlike gonorrhea, syphilis, and many other diseases, herpes is not a reportable disease within the United States, primarily because the absence of adequate treatment and control measures makes it difficult to justify any government surveillance. A governmental survey of consultations between randomly selected patients and physicians revealed an apparent ninefold increase for herpes treatment visitations between 1960 and 1979; this data supports the contention of medical authorities that herpes infections are presently in epidemic proportions within the United States.[57]

Studies reveal that a very large percentage of today's American populus has been exposed to some form of herpes virus.[16] Ninety-five percent of all blood samples taken reveal some degree of herpes antibody, indicating that the person was exposed to the virus but the the reticuloendothelial system (immune system) rejected the infection successfully.[16]

A 1979 study of the Herpes Resource Center revealed that 51 percent of herpes patients were females; 95 percent were Caucasians; 80 percent were 20 to 39 years of age; 53 percent had four or more years of college; 56 percent earned over $20,000.00 per year; and 56 percent were married to or residing with the infected partner.[58] According to the Herpes Resource Center, herpes infections among neonates is (fortunately) rare, with one case occurring for every 3,000 to 10,000 births.[58] Some medical investigators believe that herpes infection affects up to 20 percent of all sexually active adults within the United States.[54]

Infectious Etiological Agents

The family of viruses known as herpes viruses is a fascinating and diverse group of agents; herpes simplex viruses are large DNA viruses which code for approximately 100 type-specific proteins. The DNA sequence homology between HSV-1 and HSV-2 is approximately 50 percent; they are much more closely related to each other than to any other herpes viruses, which are quite different in terms of their DNA sequence homology. Restriction enzyme analysis of different isolates of herpes simplex virus have shown that just as there are thousands of different strains of *Escherichia coli*, there are hundreds of thousands of different strains of HSV-1 and HSV-2. In fact, except for distinct epidemiologic units such as sexual partners, mothers and babies, or families, nearly every person has his or her own strain of HSV.[60]

The behavior of viruses in general should not go unmentioned. They appear to be alive in the sense that they can reproduce; however, they appear chemical in nature as well in that they can crystallize into a lifeless form without any apparent requirements for lengthy periods of time. Viruses are the smallest pathogens affecting mankind; once inside the body, they invade individual cells and take control of the cell's nucleus, instructing the cell to produce virus particles.[10] The invaded cell bursts to release approximately 200 new viruses, which invade neighboring cells to replicate this process. The herpes viruses have an excellent relationship with the human organism from their perspective; following invasion, symptoms are produced for several days before the virus becomes dormant within neurons (nerve cells) to live within the host body for the infected person's entire life, with or without a recurrence of symptomology.[1,10,56] The entire family of herpes viruses appears capable of latency.[60]

Studies show that HSV-2 viral infection is responsible for 90 percent of intial genital herpes infections; 10 percent of such infections are due to HSV-1 genital infection. Genital infections with HSV-1 generally arise from oral-genital contact.[60]

Reservoir and Source of Infection

The reservoir is mankind; the source of infection is active lesions produced by the virus.

Mode of Transmission

Herpes virus hominis type 2 infections are generally acquired through vaginal or anal intercourse and/or oral-genital sexual activity. Type 1 infections are generally acquired through sexual or other intimate contact such as kissing or touching. Autoinoculation is a proven means of spread. Fomite transfer from contaminated objects such as drinking glasses or towels is possible; the herpes virus appears to be viable for at least 72 hours on towels and 4 hours upon toilet seats. However, the probability of acquiring herpes infections from such fomites is estimated at approximately 1 percent. The virus is not airborne.

The transmission risk by intimate contact appears low without the presence of active lesions; however, many authorities believe that the disease can be communicated during the prodromal period characterized by itching and tingling prior to a recurrence of herpes lesions.[57,58] A condom may cover a penile lesion and appears to be an effective barrier during the asymptomatic viral shedding period in which a male sheds the virus in his seminal fluid or a female sheds the virus from her cervix.[60] However, transmission of herpes has occurred despite the utilization of condoms; this being the case, one should abstain from sexual activity when active lesions are present and not depend upon a condom for protection.[60] The virus probably does not penetrate the condom, but often the condom is not utilized early enough, or else there may be secretions that reach the outside of the condom or lesions which are outside of the condom.[60] The virus enters the skin through a lesion or through the mucous membrane tissues and enters the nervous system nearest the site of infection, most commonly in the trigeminal or sacral ganglia.[57] Once within a nerve cell, the virus restricts itself to that area; it is not found in the blood, yet it can cause permanent damage if it results in perinatal eye or encephalitis infections.[57]

Many studies show that viral shedding may occur in the absence of clinical manifestations of disease in 1 to 10 percent of cases, depending upon the population investigated.[57] While the role of viral shedding in these low titers is idiopathic, the implications for transmission are potentially serious.[5] An important question is whether a patient with herpes should refrain from sexual contact due to fear of viral shedding and consequent transmission of disease. This dilemma to the herpes patient is devastating and real.[57]

Incubation Period

Herpes lesions generally develop within 3 to 7 days (with a range of 2 to 20 days) following infection, often beginning with a burning or tingling sensation.[54,59] The herpes sores, or fluid-filled blisters, spontaneously resolve or rupture to form shallow painful sores which then scab and heal.[1,10,57] Inguinal lymphadenopathy with tenderness is typical, with the initial herpes lesions lasting for approximately 14 to 28 days.[57,58,59,60] Although the herpes lesions disappear, the virus remains lifelong within neurons and can multiply at a later date to cause herpes lesions once again.[59] The number of herpes recurrences is highly variable, with recurrent lesions generally lasting approximately 7 to 14 days.[57,59]

Period of Communicability

Inadequate information presently exists concerning herpes infections; however, generally, the disease is believed to spread by direct contact with herpes lesions.[57,59] During the dormant period between recurrences, the individual is generally less likely to spread disease.[59] During the prodromal period characterized by burning, pruritus, and tingling just prior to recurrence of lesions, the disease may be more easily communicated than during the dormant period. However, as previously noted, numerous studies have indicated that viral shedding may occur in the absence of clinical manifestations.[60] Such incidence is low, affecting approximately 1 to 10 percent of the United States populus studied.[60] Finally, it should be remembered that the virus is believed to remain viable for up to 72 hours on a towel and up to 4 hours on a toilet seat — much longer than previously believed.

Susceptibility and Resistance

Susceptibility is general; people with herpes virus hominis infections and the virus itself are ubiquitous.[57] All immunocompromised patients are at a particularly high risk of developing infection, along with medical personnel, who are at high risk for contracting and communicating the disease.[1,57,58] The reason why some people are infected and never exhibit the disease while others exposed to the virus are subject to a lifetime of periodic recurrences remains idiopathic.[59] Studies reveal that patients with the most severe cases of herpes often have the highest antibody titers to HSV infections yet are *more likely* to have recurrent infections.[59] This is contrary to the nature of most other viral infections.

What causes a recurrent herpes infection in someone who has maintained the dormant virus for years is idiopathic;[10,59] there is no clear or apparent pattern.[55] Potential precipitating factors include sunlight, local trauma, sexual intercourse, friction, emotional stress, poor nutrition, menstruation, or anything else which results in a physiologically compromised state.[10,59] In the case of friction, it has been noted that tight jeans, jockey shorts, panties, or panty hose may precipitate a recurrence in some individuals.[10,58]

Genital HSV-2 infections are more apt to recur than are genital HSV-1 infections, although HSV-1 infections *in general* occur more frequently.[57] Studies reveal that only 30 percent of all active cases of HSV-2 are new infections; the rest are recurrences in individuals who have had the disease before.[55]

Signs and Symptoms

There are three general classifications or stages of herpes type 1 and type 2 infections: primary, initial, and recurrent. The *primary infection* is the most severe, with lesions lasting from 7 to 21 days; a primary oral infection will present with lesions in the mouth. Primary infection is diagnosed when a patient experiencing his first outbreak shows no antibodies to HSV in acute-phase serum.

Milder clinical symptoms are experienced in *initial infections*, although the lesions can still last from 7 to 21 days. When antibodies to HSV are present in the acute serum of patients experiencing the first clinical manifestations of the disease, an initial infection is indicated; a past infection has occurred, but without symptoms.[57]

Patients with *recurrent infections* have experienced previous symptoms at least once and have high antibody titers. The number of recurrences varies from patient to patient. Some may never experience a recurrence, while others may have outbreaks every few days or weeks.[57,58,59] However, there is some evidence to suggest that recurrences become progressively milder and less frequent.[57]

Studies reveal that most patients contract type 1 infections, which are generally above the waist and affect in particular the lips, mouth, nose, chin, or cheeks, especially during childhood. A rash or lesions involving the mouth and gums appear shortly after exposure; symptoms may be hardly noticeable or may necessitate medical attention for pain relief.[54,55,58] Typically, lesions present as small, clear, fluid-filled blisters, and may also occur upon mucous membrane tissues or skin wounds.[16,54] Type 2 infections generally infect the patient below the waist and only upon the genitalia; however, the type 2 virus can cause herpes lesions upon the face or head, just as the type 1 virus may infect the genitals.[16,58] Recall that only a culture can conclusively diagnose the type 1 or type 2 infection, as the viruses are clinically indistinguishable.[57]

The clinical manifestations of primary genital herpes generally involve multiple anatomic sites and cause both local and systemic symptomology. Generally within 2 to 12 days following viral exposure a lesion or cluster of lesions appear as small and painful fluid-filled vesicles (blisters) upon the sexual genitalia.[10] The number of lesions present during any given episode may vary from one to many. In women, the lesions are generally upon the vaginal lips; however, the clitoris, cervix, outer vagina, and anal region are commonly involved.[10] In heterosexual males, the lesions most commonly present upon the shaft of the penis, while in gay and bisexual males, the lesions may be upon the penis, mouth, rectum, nipple or the chest. One to several days prior to the eruption of the blisters, a *prodromal period* occurs, characterized by pruritus (itching), parasthesia (tingling), and pain or tenderness in the thighs, buttocks, or genitalia.[54] Shortly after their appearance, the blisters soon rupture to form soft and usually extremely painful open sores with an erythemic (red) base.[10,58] Upon the cervix, the lesions are generally painless and often unnoticed as they may be covered by a yellow-gray secretion deep within the body.[10] The lesions sometimes spread to the entire surface of the vaginal lips, thighs, etc.; secondary bacterial infection of exposed lesions produces a purulent exudate (pus discharge) or bleeding with inguinal lymphadenopathy and tenderness.[1,10,60] Pruritus (itching), vaginal exudate (resulting from cervicitis) and urethral exudate (resulting from urethritis) are frequently present along with fever, photophobia, malaise, and myalgias in 40 percent of cases.[60]

Females usually have twice as many lesions as males and the lesions usually last twice as long.[58,60] Uncircumcised males with penile lesions usually suffer maceration of tissue and prolonged infections due to the chronically moist nature of the skin. Moist-skin lesions will tend to heal much more slowly than those on dry skin.[57]

Herpes infections are often accompanied by dysuria (urinary pain). If urine passes over open herpes lesions, extreme pain is experienced. Edema or swelling is a common problem as well, sometimes requiring hospitalization for urinary retention.[57]

Following 4 to 5 days of presentation, herpes lesions become less painful and begin to heal spontaneously. Skin is gradually replaced beginning at the edges of the sore, with lesions healing completely with little if any scarring. Symptoms of primary genital herpes last for approximately 2 weeks, and the healing phase takes another 10 or 11 days; thus the entire bout of illness lasts for approximately 3 weeks.[60]

Herpes pharyngitis is a common manifestation of primary disease which generally follows oral-genital contact and results from either HSV-1 or HSV-2. Herpes pharyngitis affects approximately 10 percent of primary herpes patients, who present with sore throat, lymphadenopathy, fever, malaise, and tonsillar exudate; it is commonly confused with streptococcal pharyngitis. When a patient presents with both pharyngitis and dysuria, a pelvic examination should be performed to exclude or rule out the diagnosis of herpes infection.[60]

Diagnosis

The diagnosis of herpes infection can generally be made by clinical manifestations and patient history; few possibilities exist in the differential diagnosis of recurring and painful lesions within the oral or genital region(s).[1,10,57] The Communicable Disease Center notes that a presumptive diagnosis is further supported by direct identification of multinucleated giant cells with intranuclear inclusions in a clinical specimen prepared by Papanicolaou (Pap) or other histochemical stain; typical HSV morphology by electron microscopy; detection of HSV antigens by radioisotope or enzyme assays (it should be noted that immunoassays potentially may detect biologically inactive or defective viral particles); or by an increased CF or other serologic titer in convalescent serum.

The definitive diagnosis of herpes infections is by HSV viral tissue culture that demonstrates the characteristic cytopathogenic effect (CPE) following inoculation of a specimen from the cervix, the urethra, or the base of a genital lesion. The isolates can be identified as type 1 or type 2 by fluorescent antibody, neutralization, or other serological techniques.[12] Although a positive culture can be seen in 24 to 48 hours, cultures are generally held for 7 to 10 days before they are declared as negative. It should be noted that it is possible for classic herpes lesions to yield negative cultures, particularly if older lesions with low viral titers are cultured.[57] Most major cities have a virology laboratory which can grow and identify HSV, and cultures performed in rural areas will keep without any problem for 48 to 72 hours on ice for shipment to a central laboratory.

A Pap smear can be easily performed by placing a scraping of cells from the affected area upon a slide and utilizing a differential stain to visualize multinucleated giant cells. While the virus is not seen, its effects upon living cells are visible. Smear tests are highly specific (over 90 percent) for HSV so that there is little chance for a false positive reading, but their sensitivity is too variable (25–75 percent) to be relied upon for an accurate diagnosis. Similarly, a serum antibody level should not be utilized for diagnosis as it may indicate previous infection.[57]

Indirect immunoperoxidase (IIP) and direct immunofluorescence (DI) tests in our hands are about 20 percent more sensitive than the Tzanck smear; compared with tissue culture, commercially available immunofluorescence and immunoperoxidase tests detect approximately 70 percent and Tzanck smears approximately 50 percent of HSV infections. The IIP and DI tests cannot be utilized as screening procedures in most patient populations due to their poor predictive value; if one studies patients with genital herpes lesions with both the IIP and DI tests, more than 20 percent of the specimens will yield a false positive. It is hoped that monoclonal antibodies will eventually lead to better diagnostic tests for genital herpes.[60]

Treatment

The Communicable Disease Center at Atlanta, Georgia, recommends that for the first clinical episodes, clinicians may elect to use Acyclovir ointment, 5 percent, applied in sufficient quantity to adequately cover all lesions every 3 hours, 6 times a day, for 7 days. Chemotherapy should be initiated as early as possible following the onset of symptomology. The involved area should be kept clean and dry.

Acyclovir (Zovirax Ointment 5 percent), by Burroughs Wellcome, was approved by the FDA on March 30, 1982, with tests showing that it shortens episodes of genital herpes but does *not* cure herpes; the virus still remains for the life of the host.[5,60] With Acyclovir, a significant decrease in pain and healing time arises in instances of initial infection. Studies of both men and women with recurrent disease showed the drug decreased shedding of live virus during this phase; it significantly reduces multiplication of the virus and reduces the duration of pain in immunodeficient patients.[57] Thus, this form of chemotherapy is effective and is currently recommended as the treatment of genital herpes infections.[12,39]

Note that because both initial and recurrent lesions shed high concentrations of virus, patients should abstain from sex while symptomatic. An undetermined but presumably small risk of transmission also exists during asymptomatic intervals. Condoms may offer some protection. Annual Pap smears are recommended, and pregnant women should make their obstetricians aware of any history of herpes infection.[12]

The Pennsylvania Department of Public Health, Division of Acute Infectious Diseases, specifies the following treatment for herpes infections: bland ointments, Xylocaine, warm sitz baths, and oral analgesics as well as counseling for carcinoma (routine Pap test necessary), pregnancy, and recurrence. Topical Acyclovir is of modest clinical benefit for primary infections; it does not prevent recurrences and is not helpful in the treatment of recurrent disease.[12]

There is a strong placebo affect for herpes infections; 60 percent of all herpes patients improve regardless of the form of chemotherapy used.[58] There is *no known cure* for herpes infections. The following *ineffective* therapies should be noted:

1. **Vaccines** are used to *prevent* disease; no vaccine has been approved for the *treatment* of disease within the United States. Several vaccines have been tested but have been found noneffective in preventing recurrences of herpes infections. All vaccines have certain risks and should not be utilized except when the benefits clearly outweigh the risks. *Smallpox vaccine* is a live-virus vaccine with serious side effects and is not effective for the treatment of herpes. *Polio vaccine* is also a live-virus vaccine with many side effects and should be utilized only to prevent polio. It is of no value in the treatment of genital herpes infection. *BCG vaccine* is a live-bacteria vaccine utilized to prevent tuberculosis. This has been shown to be of no value in the treatment of genital herpes. *Lupidon G vaccine* is a killed strain of herpes simplex type 2, developed in Germany and utilized to treat genital herpes in several countries other than the United States. It does not prevent recurrences of genital herpes. Because of the possible risks and lack of effect, this vaccine should not be utilized to treat genital herpes infections. *Influenza vaccine* is a killed-virus vaccine utilized to prevent influenza. It is not effective for treatment of recurring herpes simplex. *Yellow fever vaccine* is a live-virus vaccine approved for the prevention of yellow fever. It is not effective for the treatment of herpes simplex infections.[61]

2. **Immune stimulants.** —Proponents of immune stimulants suggest that persons with herpes virus infections lack the proper immune defenses to combat the disease, and therefore require immune stimulation. However, no immune defect has been found in patients with recurring herpes simplex infections. *l-Tetramisole (Levamisole)* is a drug taken in pill form which was originally believed to stimulate the body's normal immune system. Studies have shown that Levamisole has no effect on either oral or genital herpes infections. Some evidence suggests that this drug can cause serious side effects. This drug is available for investigational utilization only. *Inosiplex (Isoprinosine)* is also an immune stimulant drug with the same limitations as Levamisole. There is no evidence to suggest that Isoprinosine affects the course of herpes virus infections. Side effects are unknown. This drug is available for investigational utilization only. *Interferon* is a natural substance which the body produces in response to a variety of viral infections. It can be obtained only in very small quantities and is therefore reserved for treatment of severely ill patients. It is presently being utilized in cancer research. One preliminary study was conducted on utilization of interferon for prevention of herpes simplex infections in kidney transplant patients, and it was not effective. Interferon is available only for investigational utilization.[61]

3. **Antiviral agents** are specifically utilized to treat viral infections, just as antibiotics are utilized to treat bacterial infections. There are several antiviral agents which effectively kill the herpes virus in the laboratory, but which are not effective for treatment of genital herpes. *Vidarabine (Vira-A, adenine arabinoside, Ara-A)* was approved by the FDA for utilization

in the treatment of herpes simplex encephalitis (brain infection) and eye infection. Encephalitis is treated with intravenous Ara-A, whereas eye infection is treated with a topical application of 3 percent vidarabine. Topical vidarabine is not effective for treatment of genital herpes; in fact, men treated with vidarabine had slower healing times than the untreated men. A large study of a 10 percent topical preparation of vidarabine showed that it was not effective for the treatment of oral herpes simplex infection. In summary, vidarabine is useful only for brain and eye infections with herpes simplex virus. It is not recommended for the treatment of genital or oral herpes infections. This drug is available by prescription only. *Idoxuridine or IDU (Stoxil, Herplex Liquifilm)*, both the solution and ointment forms, is effective only for treatment of eye infections with herpes simplex. Many studies show that topical application of IDU is of no value for the treatment of genital or oral herpes infection. IDU is available by prescription only. *Ribavirin (Virazole)* is a new oral antiviral agent which is not licensed in the United States. It is being studied for effectiveness in influenza and herpes zoster infections. There has been only one study in the U.S. as of 1979 in which Ribavirin was utilized for treatment of genital herpes. It was not effective in preventing recurrences of genital herpes in these patients. Because of this and the possibility of harmful side effects, this drug should not be utilized for genital herpes.

4. Other treatments found to be ineffective for herpes infections include ether, vitamins C, E, and B-12; lactobacillus tablets; diets; 2-deoxy-d-glucose; zinc; lysine; providone-iodine (Betadine); dye-light therapy; silver sulfadiazine (Silvadene); non-xynol-9; steroid creams; and dimethyl sulfoxide (DMSO, Rimso-50).[61]

Complications

1. Neonatal Infections. — The Communicable Disease Center in Atlanta, Georgia, notes with respect to neonatal infections that women who have herpes genital infections have as much as a threefold risk of spontaneous miscarriage. Herpes infection increases the risk for premature deliveries. Herpes simplex virus can cause severe disease in infected infants. If a mother is infected at 32 weeks' gestation or later, there is an approximate 10 to 20 percent chance that her infant will be infected; this risk is greatest if the infant is exposed to active infection within the mother's birth canal during delivery. Infants can also be infected while still inside the uterus, although such infections are rare. If delivered through an infected vaginal canal, a baby has an approximate 40 to 50 percent chance of being infected. The mortality rate from septicemia due to herpes in infected infants may be as high as 50 percent. Pregnant women who have had a history of herpes or who develop this infection during pregnancy should notify their obstetrical service so that precautions can be taken.[59]

Lawrence Cory, M.D., in his article entitled "The Diagnosis and Treatment of Genital Herpes" (*The Journal of the American Medical Association* **248**, no. 9 Sept. 3, 1982), noted that vaginal delivery for women with general herpes is not impossible. Cory recommends that a woman be examined for genital herpes infection when she goes into labor. A Pap smear, while not a sensitive test for viral isolation, can be done within a few hours; a negative Pap smear and the absence of other symptoms (such as lesions or evidence of viral shedding) usually suggest that a vaginal delivery is appropriate. Abdominal delivery should be considered for a woman manifesting disease activity at or near term, but even an abdominal delivery is not 100 percent effective in preventing neonatal infections.

2. Endocervical Carcinoma. The Communicable Disease Center in Atlanta, Georgia, notes the following with respect to the relationship of herpes infections to cervical cancer:[59]

> Studies suggest that herpes genital infection predisposes women to develop cervical cancer. These studies are not conclusive, however, because both diseases have similar predisposing factors: Both occur in the young sexually active groups, most commonly in females with frequent sexual intercourse at an early age, most commonly in women with many sexual partners, and some studies suggest that a herpes viral infection can induce precancerous tissue changes in cervical cells. For this reason, we caution against over interpreting these data. The following data support this relationship: More antibodies to herpes simplex virus have been found in cervical cancer patients than in control patients, indicating five times increased risk; herpes simplex antigens have been found in cervical cancer cells; and women who develop cancer of the cervix more often give a history of herpes infection than do control patients. Women who have had genital herpes infection should have a cervical cancer check (Pap smear) at least once a year. Early detection and treatment can cure cervical cancer.[59]

Elena J. Bettoli, R.N., B.S.N., Research Epidemiologist at the Center for Disease Control in Atlanta, Georgia, has noted the following in regards to the relationship of genital herpes infection to cervical cancer:[57]

> A large number of epidemiological studies have focused upon the relationship of HSV-2 infection to cervical cancer. This research has demonstrated a two-fold increase in the frequency of cervical dysplasia in women with cytologically detected genital HSV infections. Also, considering the age of the patient, the number of sexual partners, and the age of first intercourse, the epidemiological patterns of genital herpes and cervical cancer are similar.
> Perhaps the most alarming finding is that women with genital herpes infections (HSV-2) have an eight-fold greater rate of developing carcinoma in situ compared to women with no HSV-2 antibodies within their serum. But it is important to emphasize that no causal relationship has been established, only a correlation between HSV-2 and carcinoma.

In other words, it is suspected that an HSV-2 infection precedes any neoplastic changes but it is not known whether HSV-2 is responsible for the tumor in which it is found. And it is interesting to note that a similar epidemiological association has been made between Burkitt's lymphoma and the Epstein-Barr herpes virus.[58]

10. Lymphogranuloma Venereum

Lymphogranuloma venereum (LGV, lymphogranuloma inguinale, or climatic bubo) is a sexually transmitted infectious disease of the lymphatic system characterized by a small primary lesion, regional lymphadenopathy, rectal stricture, elephantiasis of the genitalia, and constitutional symptoms such as fever, chills, headache, vague abdominal pains, joint pains, and anorexia, which generally present during the progression of inguinal lymphadenopathy (lymph node enlargement of the groin).[1,6,8,10,33] Spontaneous regression of nodes does not indicate recovery. This disease should not be confused with granuloma inguinale, which is an ulcerative skin infection due to the Donovan body.[33]

Occurrence

Lymphogranuloma venereum is more common than generally believed throughout the world, but it is most prevalent in tropical and subtropical regions.[6,33] The disease is endemic in the southern United States, particularly among those of lower socioeconomic status.[6] It is more common among blacks, with the greatest prevalence among those constituting the more sexually active ages of 15 to 30 years. The disease is prevalent among the sexually promiscuous, including the gay and bisexual communities.[6,35] Sex differences for this disease are not pronounced, and the disease affects all races and social classes.[6,10,35] In 1973, 600 new cases were reported to public health authorities within the United States, in comparison to 625 new cases in 1966.[33,52] However, the incidence of this disease may yet be considerably higher than the reported number of cases. An increased incidence of disease was noted in men returning from Vietnam.[33]

Infectious Etiological Agent

The infectious etiological agent of LGV is *Chlamydia trachomatis*, a bacterium which was formerly believed to be a virus.[1,6,8,10,33,52] The Communicable Disease Center in Atlanta, Georgia, notes that *Chlamydia trachomatis* is an obligate intracellular organism (can replicate only within a living cell, as can a virus) of immunotypes L1, L2, or L3.[12] LGV results from infection with one of several strains of *Chlamydia*. Other members of the bacterial family are the etiological agents of trachoma, inclusion blenorrhea, psittacosis (parrot fever), and some cases of nongonococcal urethritis. The prevalence of LGV in Southeast Asia makes it a continued diagnostic possibility.

Reservoir and Source of Infection

The reservoir is mankind; sources of infection are lesions of infected persons.[6]

Mode of Transmission

The disease is nearly always transmitted sexually.[33] Transmission is via direct contact during sexual intercourse (oral, anal, or vaginal) and by indirect contact with articles contaminated by exudates. Children often contract the disease by contact with bedfellows and from contaminated clothing.[6,8]

Incubation Period

The incubation period for LGV can vary from 2 to 30 days.[1,6,8,10,17,33] Generally, the primary lesion appears within 7 to 21 days; if the bubo represents the first manifestation of disease, the incubation period is 10 days to several months (generally 10 to 30 days).[6]

Period of Communicability

The period of communicability for LGV is variable; it may run from weeks to years during the presence of active lesions.[6]

Susceptibility and Resistance

Susceptibility appears to be general. Immunity does not follow an attack of the disease.[6] The control and prevention of this disease largely depend upon the detection and treatment of sexual contacts.[8]

Signs and Symptoms

The initial lesion of LGV is seldom noted, as it is painless, transitory and inconspicuous. Observed lesions consist of a single, small (2 to 3 mm), shallow ulceration upon the external genitalia; the initial lesion may appear upon the glans, prepuce, vulva, vaginal walls, cervix, within the urethra, or around the anus. The lesion usually heals rapidly without leaving a scar. Contracted during oral-genital sexual activity, it can cause the tongue to blister and swell followed by cervical lymphadenopathy.[17] Approximately 2 weeks following the appearance of the primary lesion, the disease progresses into its secondary stage, characterized by pain in the anogenital region.

Following the primary lesion and the secondary stage of anogenital pain, tender lymphadenopathy occurs (within 10 to 30 days following infection), which may be either unilateral or bilateral in nature. Frequently, this lymphadenopathy represents the first noticeable manifestation of disease; it consists of matted lymph nodes that adhere to the overlying skin. Known as a "bubo," this swelling may ultimately drain through fistulous openings.[1] Lymphadenopathy may occasionally regress spontaneously.[12]

Inflammation of the inguinal lymphatics may lead to massive elephantiasis of the penis, scrotum, or vulva.[1] Secondary ulceration of the skin is associated with lymphedema.[1]

Constitutional symptoms are frequently present during the early stages of the infection, particularly during periods of lymphadenopathy. These commonly include fever, chills, headache, vague abdominal pains and aches, joint pains, anorexia, malaise; occasionally, splenomegaly and conjunctivitis may be present.[1]

Many years following the onset of infection, the patient may develop a proctitis associated with rectal bleeding and a purulent exudate. Eventually, there is scar formation, and a complete fibrous ring may develop, resulting in rectal stricture, which may necessitate a colostomy.[33] Chronic proctitis is far more common in females due to the lymphatic drainage from the vagina to the perirectal glands. Involvement of the perirectal tissue causes perirectal abscesses and subsequent ischiorectal abscesses or anal fistulas. An increased incidence of malignancy of these structures follows an infection of lymphogranuloma venereum.[1]

Pedunculated tumors of the labia or clitoris may occur in females, and polypoid or lobulated growths may develop around the anus in either sex, with chronic involvement producing scarring of the lymphatics.[1]

Severe systemic manifestations may occur in some instances such as meningoencephalitis, keratitis, cutaneous lesions, and arthritis.[33] If treatment is delayed, or if the bubo does not form, the disease progresses, and in several months to 20 or more years the following complications arise: Anal/rectal complications such as stricture; genital elephantiasis; and/or cancer.[10]

Presumptive Diagnosis*

The LGV complement fixation test is sensitive; 80 percent of the cases have a titer of 1:16 or higher. Since the sequelae of LGV are serious and preventable, treatment should not be withheld pending the laboratory confirmation.

Definitive Diagnosis*

A definitive diagnosis requires isolation of *C. trachomatis* from an appropriate specimen and confirmation of the isolate as an LGV immunotype. However, such laboratory diagnostic capabilities are not widely available.

Treatment*

Tetracycline HCL, 500 mg/p.o./q.i.d.for 14 days, is recommended. The following alternative drugs are active against LGV serotypes in vitro but have not been evaluated clinically in culture-confirmation cases: *Doxycycline* (100 mg/p.o./b.i.d. for 14 days); *Erythromycin* (500 mg/p.o./q.i.d. for 14 days); and *Sulfamethoxazole* (1 gm/p.o./b.i.d. for 14 days). Other sulfonamides can be utilized in equal dosages.

Fluctuant lymph nodes should be aspirated as needed to prevent spontaneous rupture and subsequent sinus formation.[33] Incision and drainage or excision of nodes will delay healing and are contraindicated.

The patient should return for evaluation within 3 to 5 days after therapy begins. Sexual partners of the patient should be examined for STD as early as possible. The patient should return weekly or biweekly for evaluation until the infection is cured and all lesions are healed.[12]

The late manifestations of disease such as rectal stricture and elephantiasis do not generally respond to any form of medication; thus treatment is mainly surgical.[33]

---

*From the Communicable Disease Center in Atlanta, Georgia.

11. Molluscum Contagiosum

Molluscum contagiosum is a potentially sexually transmitted infectious disease of the skin and mucous membranes caused by the *Molluscum contagiosum* virus.[12,33]

Occurrence

The disease is limited to mankind and most frequently occurs in childhood, with a worldwide distribution and occasional epidemics in children's institutions, among wrestlers, and among members of the same family.[33] It is one of the rarer forms of sexually transmitted diseases seen within the United States and throughout the world.

Etiological Agent

The infectious etiological agent is the *Molluscum contagiosum* virus, which is the largest DNA virus of the pox virus group.[12] Although the virus has not been grown within the laboratory, it has been classified morphologically upon the basis of electronmicroscopy with the pox group of viruses.[33] No cross-antigenicity with other pox viruses has yet been demonstrated.[33]

Reservoir and Source of Infection

The reservoir is mankind; the source of infection appears to be direct intimate contact with an infected person, either sexual or otherwise.[33]

Mode of Transmission

The precise mode of transmission is idiopathic. Infections have been transmitted between the genitalia during sexual intercourse and from the mouth of a suckling baby to its mother's breast.[33] Successful experimental inoculation of lesion extracts to the skin of human volunteers has been reported.[33] Autoinoculation is frequent.

Incubation Period

The incubation period for *Molluscum contagiosum* varies from 2 weeks to 2 months.[33]

Period of Communicability

Presumably, this disease may be transmitted to others while the virus is in its active state, as with herpes infections. Autoinoculation is frequent, with lesions persisting for 6 months to 1 year generally; however, lesions may persist and spread for 3 to 4 years.[33]

Susceptibility and Resistance

Susceptibility is general but probably is increased through lowered resistance, as with many other forms of sexually transmitted diseases. Susceptibility is greatest in childhood and among those who are sexually or physically intimate with a large variety of different individuals.

Signs and Symptoms

Lesions may vary in number and size, ranging from 1 mm to "giant" lesions of 1 to 2 cm in diameter—usually 1 to 5 mm, with an average of 4 mm.[12,33] The lesions are smooth, rounded, shiny, firm, flesh-colored to pearly white papules with characteristic umbilicated centers and a waxy appearance.[12,33] The lesions are elevated and most commonly appear (either alone or in groups) upon the face, especially the eyelids, as well as on the thorax and the anogenital region.[33] The conjunctiva, lips, and buccal mucosa may rarely be involved.[33] By squeezing these papules, one can express from the umbilicated central pore a curdlike, cheesy material, which, upon electron microscopic examination, prove to be loaded with MC virus particles.[33]

Spontaneous regression without scarring eventually occurs. These lesions are frequently traumatized and become secondarily infected, but injury seems to cause individual lesions to resolve.[33]

Presumptive Diagnosis*

This disease can generally be diagnosed upon the basis of a typical clinical presentation.[12]

Definitive Diagnosis*

Definitive diagnosis is by microscopic examination of lesions or lesion material which reveals pathognomonic molluscum inclusion bodies.[12] The diagnosis of multiple lesions is fairly simple; a single lesion may be confused with a keratoacanthoma, basal cell epithelioma, or pyogenic granuloma.[33] Ordinary light microscopy smears of the lesion exudate show a specific diagnostic picture of clusters of cells containing eosinophilic, giant cytoplasmic inclusion bodies.[33]

Treatment*

Lesions may resolve spontaneously without scarring; however, they may be removed by curettage after cryoanesthesia. Caustic chemicals (podophyllin, trichloracetic acid, silver nitrate) and cryotherapy (liquid nitrogen) have been successfully utilized. If every lesion is not extirpated, the condition may recur.

The patient should return for a follow-up examination within 1 month of treatment so that new lesions may be removed. The patient's sexual partner(s) should be examined and treated as necessary.[12]

---

*From the Communicable Disease Center in Atlanta, Georgia.

12. Nonspecific Nongonococcal Urethritis

Nonspecific Nongonococcal Urethritis (NSU, NGU) is any urethritis not caused by *Neisseria gonorrhoeae*, the gonococcus.[1,6,8,10,33] The term "nonspecific" denotes that at the time the disease was identified and named, its etiology was idiopathic. This is much less true today.[12,49] While less is known about NGU than some of the other forms of sexually transmitted disease, a substantial amount of scientific information now exists concerning this disease, which may be the most common but least serious of the sexually transmitted diseases in general.[13,30]

Postgonococcal Urethritis (PGU), a variant of NGU, occurs when urethritis recurs following definitive treatment for gonorrhea. In such a case, the PGU probably represents 2 or more infections of *N. gonorrhoeae* concurrent with one or more other pathogenic organisms.[34] Pathogenic microorganisms commonly associated with NGU and PGU are *Chlamydia trachomatis* and *Ureaplasma urealyticum*.[34]

Occurrence

The disease is exceedingly widespread worldwide and may represent the most common infection, or at least most common form of STD, within the United States today.[10,44] Present estimates are that approximately 2.5 to 3 million cases of NSU or NGU occur within the United States alone each year.[13,29,30] The Communicable Disease Center in Atlanta, Georgia, estimates that some 2.5 to 3.0 million Americans have NSU and that 100,000 babies born to women with chlamydia develop pneumonia or an eye infection during birth.[13] In screening 90 pregnant women for a variety of STDs at an Atlanta Hospital, CDC officials found that 24 percent had chlamydial infection.[13] During the past decade in Great Britain, NSU has become even more prevalent than gonorrhea.[44] As with gonorrhea, women appear to be asymptomatic carriers in most instances, although the infection may involve the cervix and urethra.[44] That NGU is often asymptomatic in women poses a problem in gathering adequate epidemiological data on the disease.

Infectious Etiological Agents

Nonspecific nongonococcal urethritis is not one disease, but several different diseases caused by a variety of pathogenic microorganisms and other variables.[10,12] Some of the major etiological factors for NSU identified to date include the following:[1,10,12,49]

1. Chlamydia trachomatis.—Different forms of *Chlamydia trachomatis* probably cause approximately 50 percent of all NSU cases. Once believed to be neither viruses nor bacteria, chlamydiae are now accepted as rather unusual forms of bacteria. *Chlamydia* can cause trachoma (an eye infection which may become chronic and lead to blindness), inclusion conjunctivitis of the newborn, nongonococcal urethritis, and lymphogranuloma venereum.[29]

Tests performed on urethral secretions and morning urine specimens identified the etiological agent of NSU in 143 of 164 males as follows: 59 patients (36 percent), *Chlamydia trachomatis*; 48 patients (29.2 percent), *Ureaplasma urealyticum*; 18 patients (11.0 percent), both *C. trachomatis* and *U. urealyticum*; 18 patients (11.0 percent), other causative organisms such as *Mycoplasma hominis*, enterococci, streptococci of groups A and B, enterobacteria, and trichomonas; and in 21 patients (12.8 percent) no causative organism was isolated.[49]

2. T-stain mycoplasms.—Often confused with viruses, these organisms contain both DNA and RNA and lack a cell wall which renders penicillin-like drugs (whose mode of action is the interference with cell-wall synthesis) ineffective against them.[10] Only broad-spectrum antibiotics destroy these organisms. Sherpard found T-stains in 60 to 93 percent of patients with NSU and in 21 to 26 percent of patients within his control group; thus, they do not necessarily cause disease.[10] It is possible that the organisms can cause disease only in men who are particularly susceptible to urethritis.

3. Allergic reaction.—The exudate of NSU may represent an allergic response to vaginal or rectal secretions, birth control preparations, rectal lubricants, etc.[10,35]

4. Trichomonads.—Infection of the male urethra with *Trichomonal vaginalis* produces an exudate and "tickling sensation" upon urination due to this protozoan organism, which generally does not survive well within the urethral mucosa.[10,35] The organism is a pear-shaped protozoan with 4 flagella. It also represents the etiological agent for *Trichomonal vaginalis* vaginitis, accounting for 40 percent of all vaginitis.[10,35]

5. Chemical irritations.—The exudate of NSU may sometimes represent a local irritation or inflammation of the urethral canal or meatus due to certain soaps, dyes, deodorant sprays, vaginal contraceptives, etc.[10,33]

6. Escherichia coli (E. coli) is responsible for some cases of NSU, as in rectal intercourse among both homosexual and heterosexual couples. *E. coli* is a bacterium belonging to the family Enterobacteriaceae, tribe Escherichaea.[2,8] The organism is a short, plump, gram-negative, non-spore-forming mottle intestinal bacillus almost constantly present within the intestinal canal of humans and some subhuman animals as well. Outside of the human organism, and under certain circumstances, *E. coli* is responsible for infections of the urinary tract and other systems as well as for enteritis in infants.[2] The presence of this bacillus within milk or water indicates possible fecal contamination.[2,8]

7. Impaired resistance.—Impairment of the reticuloendothelial system (immune system) by poor nutrition, poor fitness, illness, smoking, air pollution, stress, emotional upset (particularly lack of love and self-esteem), fatigue, excessive drug utilization, lack of sleep and rest, as well as other factors may impair one's resistance to disease, allowing NSU or other forms of sexually transmitted disease to express themselves.[10,50,51] NSU may be associated with gonorrhea, syphilis, chancroid, vaginitis, protozoan infections, etc., and the patient must be screened for these.[1,10]

8. Postgonococcal urethritis.—An infection of gonococcal urethritis injures the urethra, and even with antibiotic chemotherapy, some time for urethral mucosal repair is needed, during which time the urethra is more susceptible to another infection.[1,6,8,10]

Reservoir and Source of Infection

The reservoir is mankind; the source of infection represents the specific agent, most commonly *Chlamydia trachomatis* or *Ureaplasma urealyticum* within vaginal secretions.[12] *E. coli* may be responsible for a significant number of infections associated with rectal intercourse.[10] NSU may arise as an allergic reaction to saliva in instances of oral-genital sexual contact.[1,6,8,10,33]

Mode of Transmission

Sexual contact is believed to be the major means of transmission for nonspecific nongonococcal urethritis, although the disease may be acquired from fomites, as in the instance of chemical irritations.[10] The disease is rare in virgin men.[10]

Incubation Period

The incubation period for NSU is generally more variable than that of gonorrhea (7 to 28 days for NSU in comparison to 3 to 9 days for gonococcal infections, with a range of 1 to 31 days for gonococcal infections possible).[30,33]

Period of Communicability

The period of communicability is not clearly understood, but presumably the disease is communicable while the specific etiological agent is present. It is generally communicated to a susceptible host during a symptomatic period of dysuria, exudate, etc.[10]

Susceptibility and Resistance

The susceptibility to this disease may be increased by means of a gonococcal or other form of urethritis; when resistance is impaired, the possibilities for NSU are increased.[10,35]

Signs and Symptoms

There is usually an exudate (discharge), which is thin, clear, and watery in appearance and may be present only during the morning prior to urinating. In some instances, the exudate may be thick and creamy as in gonococcal infections; however, such is not the rule for this disease.[10,35]

Generally, a mild pain is experienced upon urination. There may be difficulty initiating urination as well. Frequency of urination is commonly reported with this infection.

Generalized discomfort may be experienced within the urethra, glans of the penis, testicles, perineum, and inguinal region in general.

The disease is somewhat less clearly defined in females; exudate, cervical bleeding, and cervical infections have been reported. Often, chlamydial infections in women are not suspected until they deliver babies with inclusion conjunctivitis, have chlamydial eye infections themselves, or report that a sexual partner has NSU.[30] Steady female sexual partners of men with chlamydial NGU are likely to have endocervicitis.[12]

Remember that both males and (more commonly) females may be asymptomatic for this infection.[30]

Differential Signs and Symptoms

In NSU, the exudate is typically watery, clear, and thin; it may exist only during the morning prior to urination. In gonorrhea, the discharge may be thin initially, but then typically becomes mucopurulent in nature, or thick, white, and creamy.[10,35] The dysuria experienced with gonorrhea is generally much more severe and consistent than that experienced by patients with NSU.[10,35] Gonorrhea is characterized by a shorter, more definite incubation period (almost always 3 to 9 days), while the incubation period of NSU is more variable (at 7 to 28 days).[30]

A sexual partner(s) of the NSU patient is generally less apt to be infected with NSU than is true for gonorrhea patients and their sexual partner(s).[10]

Presumptive Diagnosis*

Men with typical clinical presentations are presumed to have NGU when tests for gonorrhea are negative and they have either WBCs on gram stain of urethral exudate or sexual exposure to an agent known to cause NGU. Asymptomatic men with negative tests for gonorrhea are also presumed to have NGU if they have at least 4 WBCs per oil immersion field on an intraurethral smear. Nongonococcal endocervicitis *cannot* be diagnosed by gram stain.[12]

Definitive Diagnosis*

Definitive diagnosis is made when an agent etiologically associated with NGU is recovered from the male urethra. It must be noted that both gonococcal and nongonococcal urethritis may coexist within the same patient and that chlamydial endocervicitis can be diagnosed by culture.[12]

Treatment*

When the etiological agent is *Chlamydia trachomatis, Ureaplasma urealyticum*, or idiopathic in nature, pursue the following course of treatment:[12]

    1. Tetracycline HCL. — 500 mg p.o./q.i.d. for at least 7 days;

    2. Doxycycline. — 100 mg p.o./b.i.d. for at least 7 days.

Alternative treatment for patients in whom tetracyclines are contraindicated is Erythromycin, 500 mg p.o./q.i.d. for at least 7 days.

*From the Communicable Disease Center in Atlanta, Georgia.

Complications

When left untreated, NGU infections such as chlamydia can lead to serious complications. Men may potentially develop urethral strictures, prostatitis, and epididymitis. Women may develop sterility due to blockage of the cervix or fallopian tubes, just as in disseminated gonococcal infections. Other complications for women may include spontaneous abortion, stillbirth, and postpartum fever in pregnancy.[12,30] (see also below.)

Relationship of Chlamydia Trachomatis Infections to Pelvic Inflammatory Disease and Pregnancy

Pelvic inflammatory disease (PID) can be caused by chlamydia, gonorrhea, or both.[12] Women with chlamydial infections are typically asymptomatic until PID develops.[11] Chlamydia can also infect a newborn infant during the birth process, resulting in pneumonia or inclusion conjunctivitis.[11,12] There is also evidence that the etiological agents of NGU are associated with fetal morbidity and complications during pregnancy.[11]

  1. **Typical case presentation of PID.** — The patient may present with pain and tenderness involving the lower abdomen, cervix, uterus, and adnexae, possibly combined with fever, chills, and elevated white blood cell (WBC) count, and an erythrocyte sedimentation rate (ESR).[12] The diagnosis is more likely if the patient has multiple sexual partners, a history of PID, utilizes an IUD, or is in the first 5 to 10 days of her menstrual cycle.[12]

  2. **Presumptive diagnosis of PID.** — Women who have the typical clinical presentation are presumed to have PID if other serious conditions such as acute appendicitis or ectopic pregnancy can be excluded.[12]

  3. **Definitive diagnosis of PID.** — Direct visualization of inflamed (edema, hyperemia, or tubal exudate) fallopian tube(s) at laparoscopy or laparotomy makes the diagnosis of PID definitive; a culture of tubal exudate establishes the etiology.[12]

  4. **Hospitalization and inpatient treatment.** — Hospitalization of patients with acute PID should be strongly considered when the diagnosis is idiopathic; surgical emergencies are excluded such as appendicitis and ectopic pregnancy; a pelvic abscess is suspected; severe illness precludes outpatient management; the patient is pregnant; the patient cannot follow an outpatient regimen; the patient has failed to respond to outpatient

therapy; and/or the clinical follow-up after 48 to 72 hours of antibiotic treatment cannot be arranged.

Many experts recommend that all PID patients be hospitalized for treatment.[12]

5. Inpatient treatment of PID. — Doxycycline, 100 mg i.v., b.i.d., plus Cefoxitin, 2.0 gm i.v., q.i.d. for at least 4 days and at least 2 days after the patient defervesces. Continue doxycycline, 100 mg p.o., b.i.d. after discharge to complete at least 10 to 14 days of therapy.[12] This regimen provides optimal coverage for *N. gonorrhoeae* (including PPNG) and *C. trachomatis* but may not provide optimal treatment for anaerobes, pelvic mass, or IUD-associated PID.[12]

6. Ambulatory treatment. — Cefoxitin, 2.0 gm; or Amoxicillin, 3.0 gm p.o., or Ampicillin, 3.5 gm p.o., or aqueous procaine penicillin 4.8 million units i.m. at 2 sites (GC) along with probenecid, 1.0 gm p.o. followed by Doxycycline 100 mg p.o., b.i.d. for 10 to 14 days.

13. Pediculosis Pubis (Crabs)

Pediculosis pubis is the infestation of pubic and other hairy regions of the body with *Phthirus pubis* (the crab louse).[1,6] Common names for this infestation include crabs, cooties, lice, and lousiness.[6,35]

Occurrence

Occurrence is worldwide, with epidemic outbreaks within families, dormitories, military bases, and institutions. Sales for one over-the-counter product to treat lice have increased 1000 percent over the past 10 years, indicating the frequency of such infestation.[10] A study of seven public STD clinics revealed that pediculosis pubis is the third most common STD in men, preceded by NGU and gonococcal infections and followed by condylomata acuminata and herpes progenitalis, respectively.[14] For women pediculosis pubis is the fifth most common; the most common STD for women is gonorrhea, followed by trichomoniasis, nonspecific vaginitis, condylomata acuminata, pediculosis pubis, and herpes progenitalis.[14] Approximately 59,000 males and females sought treatment at physicians' offices for pediculosis pubis infestations in one year within the United States, with many others treated at clinics or through self-treatment with over-the-counter (OTC) preparations.[14]

Infestative Etiological Agent

Pediculosis pubis is caused by a crab louse (*Phthirus pubis*), which has 3 claws and 4 legs and looks very much like a crab under a microscope.[10,35] Generally, the "crab" infests the hairy anogenital region, but it may infest the hairs of the axillas, eyebrows, eyelashes, beard, and entire body surface.[1,6,8,10] The pubic louse moves by swinging from hair to hair; then, with its claws tightly holding onto a pubic hair, it bites its host to feed upon the blood within capillaries.[10] The louse is yellowish-gray and difficult to see upon the skin. Following a meal, it is swollen with blood and can be more easily seen as a rust-colored speck.[10]

Phthirus pubis lives a 30-day lifetime, sexually matures within 2 weeks, and mates frequently.[1,10,33] The female louse lays approximately 3 oval whitish eggs each day, an average of 50 eggs in her lifetime. She cements the eggs firmly to one side of a hair near the skin's surface.[10,35] The eggs are firm and can be more easily felt than seen; generally the eggs hatch within 7 to 9 days.[10,35] In all stages of its life cycle, the crab louse feeds upon human blood frequently; the optimum temperature for the louse is approximately 87°F.[48] Crab lice will abandon a dead person, sick individual, or someone overheated by exercise.[48] Separated from its human host, a crab louse will die within 24 hours.[10,35,48] Others forms of lice include *Pediculosis humanus corporis* (the body louse) and *Pediculosis capitus* (the head louse); "subhuman" animal lice do not feed upon humans.[6]

The biological classification for lice is as follows: kingdom—Animalia; phylum—Arthropoda (the insect vectors or hosts associated with important human infectious diseases, arthropods are elongated segmented invertebrates, possessing an exoskeleton, bilateral symmetry, and paired jointed appendages, with two classes containing the important vectors of infectious microorganisms). *Phthirus pubis* is a member of the class Insecta, which includes arthropods with a distinct head, thorax, and abdomen; 1 pair of antennae; 2 pairs of wings on the thorax; 3 pairs of legs on the thorax; and a segmented abdomen. The order is Anoplura (lice), which includes those arthropods without wings, flattened dorsoventrally, with jointed antennae and a sucking mouth.[8]

Reservoir and Source of Infestation

The reservoir is mankind.[1,6,10] The sources of infestation are infested individuals and their personal belongings, particularly clothing and bedding.

Mode of Transmission

Transmission is directly by intimate contact with an infested person, or indirectly by contact with infested items such as underclothing, bedding, toilet seats, towels, etc.[1,10,33,48] The most common means of transmission, however, is by sexual contact.[10,48] Pubic hairs to which nits or eggs are attached are often shed from the body. Larvae hatching from these eggs may be picked up from clothing, blankets, towels, etc.[11]

Incubation Period

Under optimal conditions, the eggs of the lice hatch within one week, with the lice reaching sexual maturity within 2 weeks.[1,6,10,13,46] Significant signs and symptoms generally arise within 4 to 5 weeks of infestation.[10]

Period of Communicability

Pubic lice may be transmitted to others while the lice remain alive upon the infested person or in his/her clothing, bedding, etc., and are communicable until the eggs as well as the lice themselves have been completely destroyed. Clothing not worn for 24 hours is generally safe; however, all clothing, bedding, etc., should be thoroughly washed and a disinfectant spray utilized to destroy lice and eggs upon mattresses, etc.[10,48] In order to survive, the lice must feed upon human blood within 24 hours.[10,46]

Susceptibility and Resistance

Susceptibility is general; any person may become infected under suitable conditions of exposure. There is no resistance to reinfestations. Repeated infestations often result in dermal hypersensitivity.[6] Some patients are asymptomatic for the rash and pruritus (itching) that most patients experience with this condition.

Signs and Symptoms

Itching begins and becomes increasingly more intense (and may be most intense at night); this scratching does not bring relief but instead spreads the lice. Pruritus is an allergic reaction to the saliva and excrement of the lice. Not all people are allergic, thus not all people suffer pruritus. Small, hemorrhagic spots may be seen on the front of underwear where the lice have bitten their host. Some patients experience a rash of small, sky-blue spots where bites have occurred.

Diagnosis

Definitive diagnosis is by magnifying glass or microscopic demonstration of *Phthirus pubis* as well as nits or eggs, in conjunction with clinical symptomology of pruritus, hemorrhagic spots upon underclothing, or sky-blue spots upon the skin (any or all of these symptoms may occur). Other potential causes of pruritus must be given consideration, such as concurrent scabies infestation, scratch dermatitis, etc.[1,33]

Treatment

A number of over-the-counter preparations, such as A-200, are effective in killing lice. The Pennsylvania Department of Health, Division of

Infectious Diseases, recommends Kwell (gamma benzene hexachloride) cream or shampoo. The cream should be applied after bath, from the umbilicus to the knees. This should be left on for 8 hours; then another bath should be taken. This complete procedure should be repeated within one week. Alternatively, Kwell shampoo may be applied from axillae to knees for 5 minutes; then rinse. Repeat this procedure after one week. (An allergic reaction to Kwell sometimes occurs, resembling the dermatitis of scabies, which may concurrently exist with pediculosis pubis. Careful diagnosis is important.)

Another medication recommended is RID, which should be applied to the infested region until that region is wet and allowed to remain on for 10 minutes; wash off with soap and water. The patient should not exceed two applications of RID within 24 hours. Note that RID is preferred to Kwell for the treatment of children.

If eyelids or eyebrows are involved, Vaseline should be applied twice daily to those areas for 8 days.[39]

The Communicable Disease Center in Atlanta recommends Lindane (1 percent) lotion or cream applied in a thin layer to the infested and adjacent hairy areas and thoroughly washed off after 8 hours; or Lindane (1 percent) shampoo, applied for 4 minutes and then washed off (*not* recommended for pregnant or lactating women).[12]

In addition to the treatments described above, all underclothing, bedding, and other potentially infected clothing and objects should be washed and sprayed with Lysol or R&C spray. It is important to note that ordinary soap and water *do not* kill lice.

To facilitate control of lice, children and patients in institutions should be directly inspected for infestations, and appropriate treatment and prophylactic measures be utilized. Likewise, infested persons should advise their sexual partners to treat themselves for potential infestation. Finally, the public should be educated concerning sanitation, personal cleanliness, etc., in the hope that such education will control outbreaks.

14. Pinta

An acute and chronic infectious disease of the skin caused by *Treponema carateum*. It is characterized by an initial papular lesion of the skin followed by depigmentation of areas of the extremities and hyperkeratosis of the soles and palms.[6,33] The disease is also known as mal del, pinto, azul, tina, lota, and other names.[1,6,33]

Occurrence

Pinta is found almost entirely within the Western Hemisphere and is particularly prevalent in Mexico, Columbia, Venezuela, and Ecuador.[6,33] The disease is most prevalent among blacks within the tropics and subtropics, with pinta-like conditions reported from the east and west coasts of Africa, North Africa, the Middle East, and in India and the Philippines.[6] The disease is predominately pediatric in nature.[6,33]

Infectious Etiological Agent

Pinta is caused by *Treponema carateum*, which is morphologically indistinguishable from *Treponema pallidum*.[8,33] The precise relationship of this disease to other treponematoses (syphilis, yaws, and endemic syphilis) has not been definitely determined, and there are many similarities in the clinical manifestations of these infections.[33]

Reservoir and Source of Infection

The reservoir is mankind; the source of infection is principally initial skin lesions and those of early dyschromic stage.[6]

Mode of Transmission

Pinta is generally transmitted from person to person by sexual or other intimate physical contact; it may also be spread by an insect vector.[33] Reports of venereal and congenital infectious transmission are rare.[6]

Incubation Period

The primary lesion appears within 7 to 20 days; this is followed by a secondary eruption 5 to 18 months later, with the development of late lesions after many years of untreated infection.[6,33]

Period of Communicability

The period of communicability for pinta is idiopathic, but potentially continues while skin lesions are active, sometimes for many years.[6]

Susceptibility and Resistance

Susceptibility is undefined, but is presumably general as in other treponemal diseases. The disease is rare in white people, suggesting some natural resistance but this suggestion is not distinguished clearly from factors of personal hygiene and socioeconomic status.[6]

Signs and Symptoms

1. **Primary lesion.** — Approximately 7 to 20 days following the infection, a scaling papule appears, generally upon the hands, legs, or dorsum of the feet and having a satellite bubo.

2. **Secondary eruption.** — Within 5 to 12 months of infection, a maculopapular, erythematous secondary rash appears and may evolve into tertiary lesions, the dyschromic stage, with achromic or pigmented (blue, pink, yellow, or violet) spots of variable size primarily upon the distal portions of the extremities but often including the trunk and face.[6] These secondary lesions are called *pintids*.

3. **Late manifestations of disease.** — Late lesions develop after several years and appear as vitiligoid, slate blue, or variously colored patches of the skin. The hands, wrists, knees, and ankles are commonly involved, and hyperkeratoses of the palms and soles are also seen.[33] Aortitis and spinal fluid abnormalities similar to those found in neurosyphilis have been observed in some pinta patients.[33]

4. **Potential death.** — Rarely, untreated pinta may result in death.[6]

Diagnosis

Pinta may be diagnosed by darkfield examination and STS, the latter of which become positive during the secondary rash and thereafter behave as for veneral syphilis.[6]

Treatment

A single injection of 1.2 million units of procaine penicillin or benzathine penicillin G produces rapid disappearance of the *T. carateum* from the lesions of pinta and a decline in the serologic titer. It is the treatment of choice in this disease and is more effective than tetracyclines or chloramphenicol.[33]

15. Reiter's Syndrome

Reiter's syndrome is also known as Reiter's disease, venereal arthritis, infectious uroarthritis, idiopathic blennorrheal arthritis, and arthritis urethritica and is recognized by the triad nongonococcal urethritis, conjunctivitis, and polyarthritis generally in that order.[46] Many patients also have characteristic mucocutaneous manifestations; the complete triad is not common but incomplete forms such as arthritis or conjunctivitis are frequent.[33]

Occurrence

The disease primarily affects young men, although the disease affects females and individuals in all age groups as well with a particularly high incidence in military populations.[33] In the United States and England, the disease is generally considered to be sexually transmitted in nature.

Infectious Etiological Agent

Recent reports strongly implicate a Bedsonia known as a pleuropneumonia-like organism (PPLO) isolated from joints, urethra, and eyes of several patients. In France, North Africa, and the Far East, the syndrome is sometimes considered to be a complication of bacillary dysentery.[33]

Reservoir and Source of Infection

The reservoir appears to be only mankind; the source of infection is presumably infectious exudates from patients.

Mode of Transmission

While not clearly understood, the primary mode of transmission for this disease appears to be sexual intercourse or other intimate physical contact.

Incubation Period

The triad of Reiter's syndrome generally evolves over a 3 to 4 week period, although this may vary from days to months.[33] Urethritis generally appears first, followed by conjunctivitis and then arthritis; in most instances, the arthritis is the most severe and protracted manifestation of disease.[33]

Period of Communicability

Presumably the disease is communicable while the infectious agent is present in the patient's exudates, although the actual period of communicability is unknown.

Susceptibility and Resistance

Susceptibility appears to be general, with the disease commonly associated with gonorrhea or some other form of sexually transmitted disease. The initial attack of urethritis and conjunctivitis appears to be self-limited, while the initial attack of arthritis is likely to be explosive.[33]

Signs and Symptoms

Harrison and his associates have well described the symptomology of Reiter's syndrome in *Harrison's Principles of Internal Medicine:*[33]

1. Urethritis, dysuria, and urethral exudate. — Nongonococcal urethritis is generally the first symptom to appear and may produce dysuria and exudate. The initial attack is typically self-limited; the urethritis may disappear after a few days. Recurrences are the rule, however, with as many as 8 episodes recorded for a single patient. The urethral meatus is frequently erythemic and edematous; in addition, there may be nonbacterial cystitis manifested by frequency of urination, suprapubic pain, and terminal hematuria (blood in the urine). There may also be prostatitis or seminal vesiculitis, with urethral stricture a rare complication.

2. Conjunctivitis. — Following urethritis and preceding arthritis, conjunctivitis may present. As with the initial attack of urethritis, the initial attack of conjunctivitis tends to be self-limited, disappearing after a few days or weeks.

3. Arthritis. — Migratory polyarthritis following nongonococcal urethritis and conjunctivitis comprise the complete syndrome. The initial attack of arthritis is likely to be explosive and migratory with heat, tenderness, and edema typically noted. The most commonly affected joints are the knees, ankles, metatarsophalangeal joints, and wrists, in that order. However, any peripheral joint may be involved and the disease may be nonarticular. Severe pain in one or both heels is a common complaint. Evidence of spondylitis, such as low-back pain and stiffness or tenderness over the spinous processes sometimes appears late in the disease process. Subsequent attacks of arthritis tend to have a more gradual onset than the initial attack.

4. Mucocutaneous lesions represent an important diagnostic sign and appear early, often preceding other symptoms. Such lesions appear upon the glans penis in 80 percent of cases, within the mouth in 50 percent of cases, and upon the soles and/or palms in 30 percent of cases. The penile lesions generally begin as small blebs, which coalesce into large patches with sharply defined borders (balanitis circinata). Oral lesions upon the palate, buccal mucosa, tongue, and pharynx consist of small painless papules or vesicles which coalesce to form irregular gray patches demarcated by a red serpiginous border. Lesions upon the soles and palms consist of keratoderma blennorrhagicum, beginning as hyperkeratotic red-purple papules, often in clusters, which may later coalesce.

Diagnosis

The diagnosis is by clinical manifestations of disease along with differential diagnosis of gonococcal, psoriatic, rheumatoid and other forms of arthritis as well as related syndromes.

Treatment

Treatment is purely symptomatic; mild cases require only salicylates, while the most severe cases generally respond to phenylbutazone or indomethacin with corticosteroids.[33]

16. Scabies

Scabies is a transmissible parasitic skin infection characterized by superficial burrows, intense pruritus, and secondary inflammatory changes due to a crab-shaped mite, *Sarcoptes scabiei*.[1,6] Penetration of this mite is visible as papules or vesicles with lesions prominent around the male genitalia, finger webs, anterior aspect of the wrists, anterior elbows, anterior axillary folds, belt line, thighs, nipples in women, lower buttocks, and upon the face of infants (rarely so for adults).[1,10]

Occurrence

Occurrence is worldwide and widespread; the disease is particularly common during times of war, poverty, or social upheaval. In stable times when soap and bathing facilities are ample, the infection is much less common among industrial nations; however, it remains endemic in less developed industrial nations.[6] Epidemic outbreaks are sometimes seen in households, dormitories, military bases, and institutions.[1,33]

Infectious Etiological Agent

Sarcoptes scabiei, or itch mite, is the cause of scabies; the female mite is .3 to .4 mm; the male is somewhat smaller.[12] It is the female mite that burrows under the skin to deposit eggs.[12] The biological classification for the mite is as follows: kingdom — Animalia; phylum — Arthropoda (insect vectors or hosts associated with important human infectious diseases); class — Arachnida; and order — Acarina (head and thorax fused, abdomen not segmented, no antennae, adults have 4 pairs of thoracic legs, and mouth has a hypostome, a piercing organ).[8]

Reservoir and Source of Infection

The reservoir is mankind. *Sarcoptes scabiei* live upon a human host but cannot reproduce in the skin.[6] Scabies can be contracted through contact with either vectors or fomites.[6,10,12]

Mode of Transmission

Transfer of parasites is by direct sexual or other intimate contact and, to a limited extent, from undergarments, soiled sheets, or other contaminated articles.[6] Through intimate contact and contact with contaminated articles, scabies can spread throughout a household, dormitory, military barracks, etc.[1,35] The disease may also be transmitted from cats and dogs to humans.[35]

Incubation Period

Several days or weeks may pass before pruritus (itching) is noticed.[6] An initial infection with scabies may be asymptomatic. After approximately one month, pruritus becomes apparent, and progressive in nature.[1,10,35]

Period of Communicability

The disease is communicable until the mites and eggs are completely destroyed by thorough treatment, generally after one or two courses of therapy one week apart.[6]

Susceptibility and Resistance

The susceptibility is general; anyone can become infected and reinfected any time.[6]

Signs and Symptoms

1. Pruritus becomes progressively more severe with time and tends to be particularly severe at night.

2. Erythematous/papular eruptions or lesions tend to be most prominent around the genitalia, anterior axillary fold, thighs, and elbows, belt line, nipples (in women), lower buttocks, finger webs, and rarely upon the adult face but commonly so in infants.[10,12]

3. Excoriations and secondary infections are common. —Severe pruritus results frequently in a scratch dermatitis, which makes diagnosis clinically more difficult.[1,12] Reddish-brown nodules are caused by hypersensitivity and develop one or more months following infection. The primary lesion is the burrow; when not obliterated by excoriations, it is most commonly seen on fingers, the penis, and wrists.[12]

Presumptive Diagnosis

The history, characteristic location, and appearance of skin lesions in conjunction with pruritus generally more severe at night, and the presence of similar clinical manifestations in one's sexual partner(s), make the diagnosis for scabies likely. A history of exposure to a patient with scabies within the previous 2 months supports the diagnosis.

Definitive Diagnosis

Definitive diagnosis is made by microscopic identification of the mite or its eggs, larvae, or feces in scrapings from an elevated papule or burrow.[1,10,12] If the mite is seen, the diagnosis is definitive; however, the mite is often difficult to catch, making confirmation impossible.[35] Often the diagnosis is made on clinical grounds alone.[12]

Treatment

The Communicable Disease Center in Atlanta recommends the application of Lindane (1 percent), 1 oz. of lotion or 30 gm of cream, applied thinly to all areas of the body from the neck down and washed off thoroughly after 8 hours. This drug is not recommended for pregnant or lactating women, infants, or young children.[12] Alternative therapies include Crotamiton (10 percent) applied to the entire body nightly for 2 nights and washed off thoroughly 24 hours after the second application, or sulfur (6 percent) in petrolatum, applied to the entire body nightly for 3 nights. Patients may bathe before each application.[12]

The Pennsylvania Department of Health recommends for *adults*: Bathe, then apply Kwell ointment or lotion on the entire body below the neck; wash off in 8 hours; repeat in 7 days.[39] *For infants and young children*: Bathe, then apply Crotamiton to the entire body below the neck; a second application 24 hours later; wash off 24 hours following the last application.[39] Note that Kwell allergy produces a rash that resembles scabies.

Inform sexual contacts so that they may receive similar treatment. Clothing, bedding, etc., should be carefully washed, and potentially contaminated objects sprayed with Lysol spray. Topical antibiotic chemotherapy may be essential in instances of secondary infection.[10] Psychoneurotic individuals must be assured that treatment has been definitive and as such, serves as a test-or-cure.[10]

Note that A-200, which works well on pediculosis pubis, is *ineffective* for scabies.

17. Urinary Tract Infections

Urinary tract infections may involve any part of the urinary system (kidneys, ureters, bladder, and/or urethra) and are generally caused by bacteria.[1,10]

Occurrence

Infections are most common in the age group of puberty to 45 years of age, with women much more commonly affected than men.[1,10,16] Cystitis is the most common of the many forms of urinary tract infections and may arise following vigorous and frequent sexual intercourse.[1,10,16,33] During sexual intercourse, the bladder tends to be displaced by pressure of the penis against it and the urethra through the vaginal walls.[17] The highest incidence of lower urinary-tract infections in women is within 24 to 48 hours following sexual intercourse.[17] This condition occurs frequently during honeymoons and is often called "honeymoon cystitis".[1,10,17]

Some medical authorities have specified several reasons for the much greater incidence of bladder infections in females: (1) the shorter urethra; (2) in young females, a tendency to retain urine until the bladder becomes quite distended; (3) in adults, tumors that sometimes cause urinary retention (fibroid tumors of the uterus in women, prostatic tumors in males, and bladder tumors), with resulting distention strongly predisposing to cystitis.[8] Furthermore, pregnant women may have a similar problem as the developing fetus places increasing pressure upon the surrounding pelvic structures. During labor, urinary retention is common and when catheterization is essential, another risk of infection is added to the pre-existing possibilities.[8]

Infectious Etiological Agent

Urinary tract infections frequently arise from urologic procedures performed within medical offices and hospitals, such as bladder surgery, transurethral resections of the prostate, cystoscopy, urethral or ureteral catheterizations, and the utilization of indwelling catheters for continuous bladder drainage.[8] In many instances the infection is introduced by faulty technique, unwashed hands, or inadequately sterilized equipment.[8] Many other types of diseases and anatomic problems may contribute, such as stones or tumors, which may act as focal centers for infection.

Common agents of urinary tract infections include the following microorganisms:[8] many species of gram-negative enteric bacilli, such as *Escherichia coli*, Klebsiella, Proteus, and *Pseudomonas aeruginosa; Staphylococcus aureus* and sometimes, coagulase-negative staphylococci; *Streptococcus faecalis*; and *Candida albicans* (particularly in infections of older or debilitated individuals). Infections of the lower urinary tract are often mixed, with two or more bacterial strains being synergistically active.

Authorities also note a number of pathogenic organisms associated with systemic disease that may cause primary or secondary kidney lesions and may be identified within the urine, including *Leptospira interrogans*, Salmonella species (including *S. typhi*), and mycobacterium tuberculosis.

Furthermore, the blood fluke *Schistosoma haematobium* characteristically lodges in pelvic veins, producing ova that migrate through the bladder wall and are excreted in the urine.[8]

The Merck Manual of Diagnosis and Therapy specifies the following forms of cystitis:[1]

1. Honeymoon cystitis is the term applied to bladder infections occurring in young women, generally during the first few months of marriage or sexual intercourse. Frequent and/or vigorous intercourse may cause edema of the bladder neck and urethra, impairing bladder emptying, and may predispose to the introduction of microorganisms through the urethra. Patients should be instructed to maintain a high fluid intake and to empty the bladder completely before and after sexual activity.

2. Hemorrhagic cystitis is an acute cystitis, often due to *E. coli* or streptococci. Gross hematuria is the presenting symptom, followed by frequency, urgency, and dysuria.

3. Cystitis cystica and vesicular cystitis are chronic infections with mucosal and submucosal cystic changes, similar to those observed in ureteritis cystica.

4. Cystitis emphysematosa is due to infection with gas-forming bacilli, involving the submucosal layer of the bladder wall.

5. Cystitis glandularis exhibits characteristic histologic changes of encysted epithelialized spaces beneath the mucosal lining of the bladder.

Cystitis may accompany benign prostatic hypertrophy with bladder outlet obstruction, chronic prostatitis, and seminal vesiculitis, or may initiate infection of the vasa (vasitis) and the scrotal contents (epididymo-orchitis).[1] Cystitis may have emotional as well as organic causes.[17]

Reservoir and Source of Infection

The reservoir is mankind; the source of infection is a variety of bacteria introduced into the urethra during sexual activity and particularly during times of impaired resistance.[1,10,33] Urinary tract infections also commonly arise as a result of urologic procedures, complications associated with systemic diseases, and anatomical problems of the genitourinary system.[1,8,10]

Mode of Transmission

Pathogenic microorganisms associated with urinary tract infections may be transmitted during sexual contact. Frequent sexual intercourse can result in "honeymoon cystitis" as it predisposes the bladder to infection.[1,10,33] Cystitis may arise when impaired resistance precipitates an attack of existing internal bacteria, or when infective organisms from the perineal area enter the bladder via the urethra.[1,10,16,17,33]

Urinary tract infections frequently arise from urologic procedures performed within medical offices and hospitals, such as bladder surgery, transurethral resections of the prostate, cystoscopy, urethral or ureteral catheterizations, and the utilization of indwelling catheters for continuous bladder drainage.[8] In may instances the infection is introduced by faulty technique, unwashed hands, or inadequately sterilized equipment.[8] Many other types of diseases and anatomic problems may predispose to bladder infections, such as stones or tumors, which may act as focal centers for infection.

Incubation Period

Generally, the incubation period is several days following infection. Some patients are asymptomatic for this disease.

Period of Communicability

The disease is communicable while the infective organisms are present. However, some individuals with potentially pathogenic organisms do not develop clinical disease.[1,33]

Susceptibility and Resistance

The susceptibility is general, but increased with lower resistance. Bacteria responsible for this infection are present in large numbers within the large intestine of all perfectly healthy men and women; why they infect some women and not others is unknown but presumed to be due in part to immunodeficiency.[1,10,33] Women are more susceptible than men to cystitis (see *Occurrence*, p. 143). The bladder epithelium is relatively resistant to infection, and the bladder which functions normally is not readily infected.[1] However, trauma to the bladder mucosa (stone, catheterization, instrumentation, frequent and vigorous sexual intercourse) or inadequate bladder evacuation (urinary retention, dehydration, outlet obstruction, neurogenic bladder) predisposes to the establishment of cystitis.[1]

Signs and Symptoms

Cystitis is the name by which physicians refer to urinary tract infections with pathognomonic local symptoms:[33]

1. Frequency and urgency of urination.

2. Dysuria (urinary pain) during and immediately following urination.

3. Prominent systemic symptoms. — Fever above 101°F, muscular pains, nausea, vomiting, and prostration should lead one to contact a physician. Even in the absence of systemic manifestations of infection, it is generally not possible to be certain that the infection is limited to the bladder region in cystitis patients.[1,33] Some women experience abdominal pain within the lower quandrants.[10]

4. Hematuria. — The urine may be hazy, and in some instances, tinged with blood from the walls of an infected bladder.[10] Painful intercourse is often reported.[17]

Other urinary problems and infections present as follows:

1. Acute kidney or renal infections may manifest themselves within a few hours to two days with aching pain in the lumbar region, fever which may be as high as 105°F, often with shaking chills. There may be nausea, vomiting, and diarrhea; or occasionally, constipation.[33]

2. Acute prostatitis presents as dysuria and frequency followed promptly by a severe febrile (fever) response; the prostate is diffusely swollen and tender.[1]

3. Chronic prostatitis may follow an acute prostatic infection or may develop insidiously to produce symptoms of minor urinary irritation, including frequency, nocturia (need to urinate at night), and dysuria; the prostate may be moderately tender and boggy.[1]

Diagnosis

Diagnosis should take into consideration the chief complaint and presenting signs and symptoms; the patient's personal and family medical history; urine and urethral culture and sensitivity; and other laboratory procedures as indicated (ultrasound, x-rays, blood work-ups, etc.).

Treatment

Gantrisin 1 gram (2 tablets of .5 gm each) p.o./q 6 hours for 10 to 24 days. Symptoms generally disappear soon after treatment. Ampicillin and other antibiotics may be prescribed depending upon the nature of the etiological agent.[10]

Females with repeated bladder infections should have a complete examination of the urinary tract by a urologist. Some women develop chronic cystitis, which requires long-term and low-dosage antibiotic chemotherapy.

18. Vaginitis

Review of the current literature and classifications utilized by the Communicable Disease Center in Atlanta, Georgia, and the Pennsylvania Department of Public Health, Division of Acute Infectious Diseases, reveals four major classifications of vaginitis:

- *Candida albicans vaginitis (candidiasis).*
- *Gardnerella vaginale vaginitis* (formerly known as Corynebacterium vaginale vaginitis, formerly known as Haemophilus vaginitis).[52,53]
- *Nonspecific vaginitis.*
- *Trichomonal vaginalis vaginitis (trichomoniasis).*

Candidiasis

Candidiasis or moniliasis is an infectious fungus disease with a variety of forms, chiefly affecting females in the cutaneous, mucosal, or systemic tissues.[1,11] *Candida albicans* and other species of candida cause a fungus infection characterized by vulvovaginitis in women, balanitis in men, oral thrush, and infection of the fingers.[1,6,10,33]

Occurrence

The occurrence of candidiasis is universal; epidemics have appeared, although the disease is generally sporadic.[1,6] Infants, debilitated persons, persons with poor-fitting dentures, those who sweat excessively or whose hands are commonly in water, those with diabetes mellitus, those pregnant, those taking broad-spectrum antibiotics, and lactating women are more susceptible to this disease, characterizing a population at risk.[1,6,10,33] Those with hypoparathyroidism or impaired reticuloendothelial systems, along with those taking Flagyl in dosage utilized to treat trichomoniasis are more susceptible to this disease.[52] Vaginal colonization is more frequent among women utilizing the oral contraceptive than among those who do not; however, the frequency of symptomology among colonized women does not appear to be increased.[52]

Vaginitis

The overall incidence of candidal genital infection in the United States is idiopathic.[52] The disease is most common in populations exhibiting a high prevalence of other sexually transmitted diseases.[52,53]

Although there is no well-documented increase in maternal perinatal morbidity in the presence of monilial infection, the rate of neonatal thrush is estimated to be approximately 3 times higher in the offspring of infected mothers.[52]

Infectious Etiological Agent

The infections are caused chiefly by *Candida albicans* (*Monilia albicans*) but sometimes other species of Candida; oral thrush rarely may be caused by Saccharomyces.[6,8] The fungus is found in fowl, other animals, and fruit.[6,8] *Candida albicans* is part of the normal flora of the mouth, gastrointestinal tract, and vagina of 25 to 50 percent of normal women.[53] The factors which allow this usually harmless saprophyte to cause symptomatic vulvovaginitis and other infections are obscure; such factors may be related to the availability of glycogen.[10,52]

Candida albicans is a dimorphous fungus; in the saprophytic state, it appears only in the yeast form with clusters of spherical blastospores. In disease due to Candida species, both yeast and mycelian forms should be seen.[52]

Reservoir and Source of Infection

The reservoir is mankind; the source of infection is secretions from the mouth, skin, vagina, and especially feces from patients or carriers. The organism also occurs on fruit and in sea water.[6,8] The organism can survive under the foreskin of an uncircumcised male.[10]

Mode of Transmission

How the disease is acquired is largely unknown, even though a number of factors have been isolated that increase one's susceptibility (see *Susceptibility and Resistance,* p. 150).[1,6,10,33,52,53] The disease is almost certainly transmitted by contact from mother to infant during childbirth and by endogenous spread.[6] The rate of neonatal thrush is 3 times higher in offspring of infected mothers. Evidence of sexual transmission of the infection is scanty.[52] However, the peak incidence for the disease coincides with the ages for maximum sexual activity (16 to 30 years of age), and Candida is frequently cultured from the urethras of sexual partners of infected women.[52] Men are more likely to acquire the disease sexually, and may in turn reinfect their sexual partners.[53]

Incubation Period

The incubation period is variable; 2 to 5 days for thrush infections in infants.[6] Symptomology is typically of abrupt onset; however, in contrast to trichomoniasis, it generally begins *before* menstruation.[52]

Period of Communicability

Presumably the disease is communicable for the duration of the infectious exudate or lesions.[6] Differentiating candidal colonization from true candidal infection of the vagina can be difficult, as *Candida albicans* is found in vaginas of 25 to 50 percent of healthy women.[52]

Susceptibility and Resistance

Inapparent infections are common. The fungus is frequently found in patients receiving antibiotic chemotherapy for lung infections and in patients with lung cancer. Many adults are hypersensitive to the fungus and possess antibodies.[6,8] Second attacks are common; clinical manifestations are likely to follow general or locally lowered resistance.[6,8,10,52]

The following factors appear to increase susceptibility:[1,6,8,10,52]

1. Pregnancy. — Changes in hormonal levels during pregnancy cause vaginal cells to store more sugar than usual within these cells, predisposing the patient to candidiasis.[10]

2. Diabetes mellitus. — Females with diabetes mellitus store greater amounts of glycogen within their vaginal cells, making them more susceptible to a potential infection.

3. Birth control pills. — Women who were initially put on birth control pills with an estrogen dosage in excess of .05 mg per pill were more susceptible to infection; the lower-dosage pills do not cause this effect.[10]

4. Antibiotic chemotherapy. — Treatment of bacterial infections with tetracycline HCL, Flagyl, etc., has no effect upon treating this infection; rather, such reduces the number of other microscopic organisms normally present within the vaginal canal. With competition reduced, Candida can multiply rapidly.[1,10,33,52] The utilization of corticosteroids has a similar effect.[53]

5. Oral diseases or ill-fitting dentures predispose to thrush.[1]

6. Frequent exposure to water. — Individuals engaged in occupations involving maceration of the skin through frequent soaking in soapy water are most apt to develop skin infections.[1,6,8] The infection in this population is often called "bartender's itch" or "housewife's itch."

7. Severe diaphoresis is particularly common in obese patients and makes candida skin infection more likely.[1,10]

8. Lower resistance. —Patients with immune deficiencies such as those with leukemia, those having organ transplants, those debilitated by poor nutrition, those under great stress, those who smoke, and those exposed to heavy pollution are at risk for candida infections.[1,10,52]

9. Nylon underwear. —Wearing nylon underwear or panty hose instead of cotton increases the temperature of the vaginal environment and creates more of an anaerobic atmosphere, which makes the vaginal pH more alkaline.[52,53] This environment favors candida infection.[1,10]

The infrequency of clinical disease suggests that host susceptibility is probably a more important factor than is degree of infectivity or communicability for this disease.[6]

Signs and Symptoms

In males, dysuria and exudate may occur along with a cheesy secretion from under the prepuce of uncircumcised men.[39] Symptomatic urethritis and frank balanitis occur in up to 10 percent of infected men.[52]

Most women who have this infection are asymptomatic. The symptomatic patient generally complains more of severe pruritus of the vulvular region than of vaginal exudate.[53] Pruritus may be severe enough to interrupt sleep and other activities. There may be a characteristic odor of fermentation.[10] The classic physical findings, present in a minority of patients, include edema of the labia minora, white patches on the vulvar and vaginal mucosa, and a thick, white, curdlike exudate (resembling cottage cheese) from the vagina.[1,10,52,53] The sexual partners of infected women may develop balanitis or cutaneous lesions on the shaft of the penis.[53] There may be dyspareunia (painful sexual intercourse). The onset of infection tends to be premenstrual in contrast to trichomonal vaginalis vaginitis.[39] The exudate may be meager if present at all.[52]

Diagnosis

Wet mount, KOH prep and gram stain should be used for both males and females. The organism may be cultured on several different antibiotic-containing media, but a positive culture alone does not make the diagnosis. A large proportion of women with vaginitis of any etiology may have small numbers of Candida among their vaginal flora.[52] Microscopic examination of the exudate allows the observer to detect the presence of yeast forms and pseudohyphae and to estimate the quantity of the fungus which is present. A small amount of vaginal exudate may be mixed with saline on a slide and observed under 400 to 1000X with the substage condenser racked down or the substage diaphragm closed down to increase contrast.[52] The overall sensitivity of the wet mount is estimated to range from 40 to 80 percent.[52]

The organisms may also be seen upon gram stain; they appear as dense, gram-positive ovoid bodies with an axis of 2 to 5 u. Pseudohyphae are long, gram-positive tubes with a diameter about the same as that of the yeast form. They may appear clear with gram-positive dots. The sensitivity of the gram stain is higher than that of the wet mount, running from 70 percent to almost 100 percent.[52]

The Pap smear is insufficiently sensitive in the diagnosis of candidiasis for routine utilization; it reveals organisms in 20 to 46 percent of culture-positive patients.[52]

Diagnosis upon clinical grounds alone is generally unreliable; it requires both a suggestive clinical picture and demonstration of the organism.[52] While there is sometimes an association between the numbers of organisms in the exudate and the severity of signs and symptoms, patients with severe symptoms may on occasion have relatively few organisms within the vaginal exudate, which increases the difficulty of differentiating colonization from infection.[52]

Treatment

1. Male (Candidiasis Urethritis). — Nystatin ointment applied to the glans of the penis and prepuce b.i.d. for 7 days.[39] Symptomatic balanitis should be treated with Nystatin cream.[10,52]

2. Female (Vaginitis). — Nystatin vaginal suppositories 100,000 u/b.i.d. for 10 days, or miconazole cream daily for 10 days,[39] or Clotrimazole, 1 vaginal suppository daily for 7 days (100 mg often recommended at bedtime). Clotrimazole is recommended for pregnant females by the Communicable Disease Center.[12] The female should wear a sanitary pad to protect clothing; suppositories should be stored within a refrigerator; and medicine should be continued during the menstrual period. The patient should refer his/her partners for clinical and laboratory evaluation and return if the problem is not cured or if it recurs. Condoms should be utilized to prevent reinfections.[12]

Symptoms of infection generally disappear within 2 days; however, the full course of treatment must be continued. Some authorities recommend that if symptoms persist in the female, Nystatin should be taken orally to destroy Candida within the large intestine and reduce the danger of reinfection.[10]

During pregnancy, candida infections may be more difficult to treat definitively. Nonpregnant women who have candida infections should be screened for potential diabetes mellitus.

If genital pruritus is severe, sitting in a tub of cool water will bring some relief; cold wet compresses may be applied to the vulva as well.[10]

Treatment Failures and Recurrences

Treatment failure or recurrence of infection should prompt an immediate and scrupulous search for predisposing factors.[52] Some cases may require replacement of oral contraception by another form of fertility control. Avoidance of restrictive or insulating clothing such as pantyhose is recommended upon theoretical grounds.[52] Combining vaginal therapy with oral Nystatin may treat a rectal focus and prevent endogenous reinfection.[52]

As the contribution of sexual transmission to the total incidence of vulvovaginal candidiasis is idiopathic, the necessity for simultaneous treatment of the asymptomatic male sexual partners of infected women is undocumented.[52] In refractory vaginal infections, culture of the male partner's urethra may reveal asymptomatic carriage, and the temporary utilization of a condom is recommended.[52] Rarely, untreated candidiasis can cause eventual damage to the heart, kidneys, and brain.[12]

Gardnerella Vaginale Vaginitis

Gardnerella vaginale vaginitis, also known as Haemophilus vaginalis or Corynebacterium vaginale, represents a superficial vaginal infection which is sexually transmissible and is characterized by a homogeneous gray or lightly colored vaginal exudate without pruritus (itching).[12,52,53] Gardner and Dukes reported in 1955 that in more than 90 percent of patients studied with nonspecific vaginitis, the infectious agent was a small gram-negative bacillus known as *Haemophilus vaginalis*.[12,52,53] Many investigators have now confirmed that this is in fact the etiological agent for this disease.[53]

Occurrence

The true frequency of this disease is idiopathic, with many case studies characterized by poor case definition and a lack of suitable controls.[52] Some authorities consider gardnerella a form of nonspecific vaginitis, while others classify the latter separately.[12,52,53] A major source of confusion concerning the etiological significance of this disease is due to its variable frequency of identification in populations of asymptomatic and diseased patients.[52] Among women with vaginitis, the agent has been isolated by culture in various studies in 23 percent, 42 percent, 47 percent, 92 percent, and 96 percent of instances.[52,53] The frequency appears to depend heavily upon the population investigated. If all women with vaginitis are cultured, the positive rate is quite low; if the survey is restricted to patients with symptoms of gardnerella vaginale vaginitis, the rate is high indeed.[52] As with trichomonas and candidiasis, the organism is also recovered from asymptomatic women at rates ranging from 0 percent to 52 percent of patients.[52] The existence of an asymptomatic carrier state is not a strong argument against the significance of the organism.[52] The organism has been postulated as an infrequent cause of nongonococcal urethritis in males. The disease is particularly common in populations at high risk for other forms of sexually transmitted diseases and may be more common in warm climates.[52,53]

Infectious Etiological Agent

The etiological agent for Gardnerella vaginale vaginitis is *Haemophilus vaginalis*, a gram-negative bacillus sometimes referred to as *Corynebacterium vaginale*.[52,53] It is generally felt by medical authorities that *Corynebacterium vaginale* is a major cause of vaginitis not attributable to Trichomonas, Candida, or other bacteria.[6,8,10,52,53] The disease has been reproduced by inoculating pure subcultures of the organism into the vagina of volunteer subjects.[53]

Reservoir and Source of Infection

The reservoir is mankind; the source of infection is vaginal and urethral exudates from infected individuals.[10,52,53]

Mode of Transmission

The disease appears to be transmitted largely by sexual intercourse, and possibly by contact with contaminated fomites.[6] Over 90 percent of sexual partners of women who have this form of vaginitis have been found to carry the infectious organisms within the urethra.[52]

Incubation Period

Incubation period is variable, but probably 4 to 20 days, generally 7 days (as for trichomoniasis).[6]

Period of Communicability

The disease is communicable for the duration of the infection, just as for other forms of vaginitis.[6]

Susceptibility and Resistance

Data suggest that some host factors are highly important in determining whether a woman will reject the organism, support it in asymptomatic carriage, or develop a chronic vaginitis.[52] Reinfections have been noted when both sexual partners are not properly treated for this disease concurrently.[52,53]

Signs and Symptoms

The patient typically presents with a gray homogeneous vaginal exudate which is generally malodorous. The exudate tends to be less voluminous than that of trichomoniasis.[10,53] Onset of the exudate is not related to menstruation.[52] Pruritus is generally absent, in contrast to other forms of vaginitis.[52,53] Studies indicate that slight pruritus or mild dysuria is reported in less than half of all infections.[52] Mild diffuse vaginitis generally exists, although punctate hemorrhages have been reported in 10 percent of patients.[52] Mild abdominal pain is frequent; however, frank dyspareunia (painful sexual intercourse) is distinctly rare.[52] Vulvar irritation is less common than in candidiasis or trichomoniasis; minimal erythema (redness) occurs in approximately 20 percent of female patients.[52]

It should be noted that approximately 10 to 40 percent of culture-positive women are completely asymptomatic.[52]

Diagnosis

Utilize a gram stain. The clue cells are epithelial cells studded with small gram-negative rods. Exudate from the vagina, *not* the endocervix, should be examined.[39]

Treatment

Ampicillin 500 mg/p.o./q.i.d. for 7 to 10 days; or triple sulfa cream or vaginal tablets (or AVC cream or suppositories) b.i.d. for 7 to 10 days.[39] Alternative treatment is Flagyl 250 mg/t.i.d. for 7 days; this may be the most effective form of chemotherapy, but there are theoretical objections to its utilization, particularly during pregnancy.[39]

Nonspecific Vaginitis

Interestingly enough, nonspecific vaginitis has by the definition of some medical authorities included Gardnerella vaginale vaginitis (q.v.), formerly known as Corynebacterium vaginale vaginitis and before that as Haemophilus vaginalis.[52,53] Gardner and Dukes reported in 1955 that in more than 90 percent of their patients with nonspecific vaginitis, the infectious etiological agent was a small, gram-negative bacillus (bacterium) known then as *Haemophilus vaginalis*, then as *Corynebacterium vaginale*, and now as *Gardnerella vaginale*.[52,53] It is generally felt that this organism is responsible for a significant number of cases of vaginitis not due to Trichomonas, Candida, or other bacteria.[52] Other studies note that the organism has been cultured in 23 percent to 96 percent (depending upon the study) of women with vaginitis.[52] Like Trichomonas and Candida, the organism is also recoverable from asymptomatic women at rates ranging from 0 percent to 52 percent.[52] The existence of a strong carrier state is not a strong argument against the significance of the organism.[52]

Diagnosis

No specific pathogens are seen or cultured.

Treatment

Nitrofurazone vaginal cream or suppositories b.i.d. for 7 to 10 days, or AVC cream b.i.d. for 7 to 10 days, or Ampicillin 500 mg/p.o./q.i.d. for 7 to 10 days.[39]

Trichomoniasis

Trichomoniasis is caused by the flagellate protozoan *Trichomonas vaginalis*; it is usually sexually transmitted and may present as vaginitis in women and, occasionally, as a form of nongonococcal urethritis in males.[53]

Occurrence

Trichomoniasis may be the most frequently acquired sexually transmitted disease among women next to gonorrhea.[53] An estimated 2.5 to 3 million cases occur annually within the United States alone.[11,30,52,53] The prevalence of positive cultures ranges from 3 to 15 percent among asymptomatic women from private practice up to 50 to 75 percent among prostitutes.[52] The prevalence among women attending gynecology clinics is 13 to 23 percent.[52] Peak incidence is between the ages of 16 and 35 years, the ages for peak sexual activity. The highest incidence is found in populations at high risk for other forms of STD; indeed, half of all women in England presenting with gonorrhea also have trichomoniasis.[52] It is estimated that at least 927,000 United States women receive treatment from a private physician each year due to this infection alone.[14] Trichomonal vaginalis vaginitis is the most common form of vaginitis in women, accounting for approximately 40 percent of all cases.[10] Some medical experts note that the disease will ultimately afflict 25 percent of all women.[17] Colonization rates are generally lower among men than among women.[6,53]

Infectious Etiological Agent

Of the many members of the genus Trichomonas, three are parasites of mankind: *T. hominis* in the intestine, *T. tenax* within the oral cavity, and *T. vaginalis*, the only one capable of producing vaginitis and urethritis.[33] All three possess 4 anterior flagella, and their morphology is quite similar (*T. vaginalis* is the largest). Confusion in diagnosis is rare due to the anatomic specificity of their habitats.[33]

Trichomonas vaginalis is a one-celled, pear-shaped protozoan slightly larger than polymorphonuclear neutrophiles; at 400X, the flagellum and the undulating membrane of viable parasites may be observed.[52] After they die, the trichomonads round up and are impossible to differentiate reliably from white blood cells.[8,52] Thousands of these organisms can be visualized microscopically within a drop of vaginal secretion.[17] Some studies indicate that the organism can survive for an entire 24-hour period when moisture is present.[10]

Reservoir and Source of Infection

The reservoir is mankind; the source of infection is vaginal and urethral exudates from infected persons.[6,8] Trichomonads house themselves under the foreskin of a man's uncircumcised penis and in severe cases may also invade the prostate; some 15 percent of men seeking treatment for urethritis present evidence of being infected with trichomonads.[17] Exactly where these organisms originated and precisely how they are contracted is not clearly understood in all instances.[17] Many gynecologists note the similarity between the trichomonads of the vagina and those found within the human intestine; however, most parasitologists maintain that the two types are actually quite different.[17] Trichomonads can survive upon wet sponges for several hours (some studies say 24) and within urine for 24 hours.[10,52] It is thus possible that transmission between adults can occur in communal settings for bathing; the spread from infected mothers to female infants during routine child care has been noted.[52]

Mode of Transmission

The sexual transmission of trichomoniasis is well established; however, like gonorrhea (and to a much easier degree), trichomoniasis can be transmitted in the absence of sexual contact.[52] In males, the organisms can enter the urethra and migrate upward to the prostate gland. As 60 percent of the male ejaculate comes from the prostate, the organisms are readily deposited within the cervix during orgasm.[16] Many scientists believe that the organism can be easily contracted from a swimming pool, bathtub, washcloth, etc. A 20 percent incidence of infection has been noted among women isolated from sexual contact within mental institutions.[17] Trichomoniasis is easily transmitted by homosexual lovemaking.[17]

Incubation Period

Experimental and clinical evidence suggests that the incubation period is 4 to 28 days.[1,10,33,52] The acute onset of pruritus (itching) and discharge often coincides with or immediately follows menstruation, and preexisting symptoms may be exacerbated at this time.[52] It is theorized that the normal acidity of the vagina is reduced by the buffering capacity of menstrual blood and that during menstruation, the pH of the vaginal milieu approaches the optimum for trichomonads (6.0-6.5) and the parasitic load increases acutely.[52]

Period of Communicability

The period of communicability is for the duration of the infection.[6] It is possible for a couple to pass these parasites back and forth for many years, particularly in the case of the male, who is commonly asymptomatic.[17] If a male wears a condom while engaging in sexual activity for 3 to 4 months, the parasites will most likely die and reinfection will end. Nothing is accomplished by curing one sexual partner only to be reinfected by the other; careful examination reveals that 60 percent of husbands of infected women have the infection.[17]

Susceptibility and Resistance

Susceptibility is general and of high grade, but clinical disease exists mainly in females.[1,6,10]

Signs and Symptoms

Males are often asymptomatic for this infection.[1,10,13] There may be exudate, dysuria, and frequency characteristic of NSU.[10,39] Many males report a slight watery exudate, mild dysuria, and a "tickling sensation" or itching within the penile urethra. The trichomonads may be under the foreskin or within the urethra itself.[10] Since fewer than 5 percent of men with nongonococcal urethritis have urethral cultures which contain *T. vaginalis*, this organism can account for only a small portion of cases of NSU.[53]

The symptoms for females are as follows:

1. Some are asymptomatic. — At least one-half of all women who are colonized for *T. vaginalis* have no symptoms; further, in one study in which consecutive OB-GYN patients were examined, more than 25 percent of colonized women had no evidence of vaginitis upon physical examination.

2. Exudate. — Classically, trichomonal vaginalis vaginitis is characterized by an abundant, watery, frothy, white, yellow, or yellow-green exudate.[10,52,53]

3. Odor. — There is a characteristic "mushroom-like" odor produced by this infection.[10]

4. Pruritus. — Severe itching of the vaginal orifice is common to this disease.[10]

5. Erythema and edema. — There is typically slight erythema (redness) of the labia minora and lower vagina, and a red-speckled appearance of the cervix and vaginal fornices.[53] Patients may suffer dyspareunia (painful sexual intercourse) and a feeling of fullness in the genitalia due to vulvar edema (swelling).[52]

6. Dysuria. — Painful urination accompanies the infection in approximately 20 percent of cases. While frank abdominal pain or rectal tenderness is rare, some patients complain of dull and poorly localized abdominal pain within the lower quadrants, which disappears when the infection is eradicated.[53]

Diagnosis

In males, a wet mount from urethral swab or exudate or a wet mount upon urine sediment is the suggested technique.[39] In females, use a wet mount from the posterior vaginal fornix.[39]

Direct microscopic examination of exudate represents a rapid and reliable method for the diagnosis of trichomoniasis.[52] A small amount of exudate is mixed upon a microscope slide with a drop of warm saline, a cover slip is applied, and the preparation is scanned under the microscope with the low or high dry objective.[53] Since active motility is necessary for identification, the slide should be examined as soon after the preparation as possible.[52] Trichomonads are revealed spectacularly by phase or darkfield microscopy.[52]

Data on 600 patients from several studies indicates a sensitivity for the wet mount of 76 percent and for the culture of 91 percent.[52] One would expect a positive culture in patients with such small numbers of organisms that the wet mount is unrevealing; direct microscopy can occasionally identify trichomonads in patients from whom a culture is negative.[52,53] Trichomonads may be cultured utilizing a variety of liquid and semisolid media, and cultures may become obviously positive within 48 hours.[52] Cultures will detect small numbers of organisms, but due to the doubling time for the parasites (a long 8 to 12 hours), cultures must be observed for 10 to 12 days before they can be reliably regarded as negative.[52,53] Trichomonads are rarely found by culture of the endocervix, and wet mount of material taken from the endocervix is likely to be negative in the presence of infection.[52]

When the wet mount technique is negative, organisms may be sometimes identified by utilizing a cytologic stain, such as giemsa stain. A smear of vaginal exudate is heat-fixed and stained for 20 minutes in routine hematologic giemsa stain. After washing briefly in tap water, the slide is examined at approximately 1000X. Trichomonads have dense blue cytoplasm and the nuclei and flagella are reddish in color.[52] Parasites are more easily distinguished from neutrophiles in this preparation than with the gram stain.[52,53]

Although trichomoniasis is sometimes diagnosed upon the basis of endocervical cytology, the Pap smear technique is unreliable, with a sensitivity range of approximately 60 to 80 percent.[52] Furthermore, the Pap smear offers no advantages over the wet mount or culture techniques.[52] Of 1,200 patients studied, the cytologic smear agreed with the results of the wet mount and culture in only 58 percent. This lack of sensitivity may relate to the infrequency with which trichomonads are found in the endocervix; the lack of specificity of the cytologic smear may result from the degree to which inflammatory cells resemble trichomonads.[52]

Differential Diagnosis

William M. McCormack, M.D., of the United States Public Health Service, author of *Practice of Medicine*, has noted five considerations which make the evaluation of a woman with vaginitis a challenging clinical problem:[53]

1. Most normal women have a physiological vaginal exudate, and the examiner must be certain that the patient who presents because of vaginal discharge actually has vaginitis. A physiologic vaginal discharge is characterized by absence of vaginal or vulvar irritation, has a normal texture and odor, and has generally been present for a long period of time. Protection with a tampon or a sanitary napkin is seldom necessary.

3. There is often considerable discordance between the patient's description of her symptoms and the findings upon physical examination.

3. The classic clinical descriptions of vaginitis are seldom seen; even when they are seen, they are not pathognomonic.

4. The organisms which have been associated with vaginal and cervical infections (gonococci, trichomonads, yeast, and *Corynebacterium vaginale*) can all be isolated from women who have *no evidence of vaginitis or cervicitis.*

5. Simultaneous colonization with more than one of these organisms is not at all infrequent.

Treatment

For males, Metronidazole (Flagyl) 2 gm/p.o. times one. For females, Flagyl 2 gm/p.o. times one. This regimen is effective, but there are objections to the utilization of this drug during pregnancy or lactation.[39] For pregnant females, Clotrimazole 100 mg intravaginally at bedtime for 7 days may produce symptomatic improvement and some cures.

Most cases of "incurable" trichomonal infections are not trichomonal infections at all.[10] Metronidazole will not cure any form of vaginitis other than trichomonal vaginalis vaginitis.[10]

Metronidazole (Flagyl) is the drug of choice for trichomoniasis. Studies indicate that a single dosage of 2 gms is comparable to 250 mg, 3 times per day for 10 days; vaginal medication is not required, although it can provide symptomatic relief.[52] A single course of treatment is at least 80 percent effective; treatment failures generally respond to a second treatment with Flagyl or are due to other organisms.[52] The patient's sexual partners should be treated simultaneously to reduce the treatment failure rate resulting from exogenous reinfection.[52]

19. Venereal Syphilis (*Lues Venerea*)

"He who knows syphilis, knows medicine" — Sir William Osler

Venereal Syphilis is an acute and chronic relapsing treponematosis characterized clinically by a primary lesion (chancre); a secondary eruption involving skin and mucous membranes; long periods of latency; and later lesions of skin, bone, viscera, and the cardiovascular and central nervous systems.[6] Two distinct forms of syphilis are recognized. Venereal syphilis, spread by sexual contact, is worldwide and the third most common reported communicable disease in the United States today.[31,34] Endemic syphilis, or bejel, is of nonvenereal spread and is confined to parts of the world where economic, social, and climatic conditions favor its development; it does not occur within the United States.[1,6,33]

The origin of the word "syphilis" dates back to 1530, when an Italian pathologist named Hieronymus Fracastorious published a poem (which achieved wide popularity) describing a shepherd named Syphilis, who had been stricken with a disease that until then had been known as "the great pox."[11,17] The disease has been known as venereal syphilis since that time. Common street names include *the pox, a pox, lues, bad blood*, and *siff*. Syphilis has also been referred to as "the great imitator" because it produces symptoms similar to psoriasis, infectious mononucleosis, a variety of skin rashes, cancer, and many other conditions.[1,10,33]

History

Despite all efforts to date, the exact origin of syphilis remains idiopathic.[1,11,17] Historically, nations have placed the blame upon one another; the English call syphilis "the French disease," and "the Spanish pox"; the French call it "the Naples disease"; and both the French and the Spanish call it "the Russian disease." For nearly 500 years, scholars and medical historians have debated the origin of syphilis, with the dispute centering around the Columbian Theory and the Pre-Columbian Theory.[10,11,17,44] The Columbian Theory proposes that syphilitic infection was well established in Hispaniola (Haiti) and was subsequently contracted and carried to Europe by Columbus's crew when they returned to

Spain in March of 1493, following their second voyage.[11,44] The Pre-Columbian Theory maintains that syphilis was present in Europe prior to the voyage of Columbus and was either unrecognized or confused with other forms of disease such as leprosy or existed in milder form.[10,11] This latter theory, also known as the "Evolutionary Theory," maintains that syphilis was not a disease in itself originally, but rather a general form of treponematosis, a "brother/sister" disease of yaws, pinta, and endemic syphilis.[10] It is believed that yaws occurred first, affecting prehistoric civilization, with the eventual evolution of venereal syphilis from these other forms.[10] Study of bones of American Indians has revealed evidence that syphilis existed in America at least 500 years before Columbus's voyages.[17]

Irrespective of origin, there is no question that a great syphilitic epidemic suddenly appeared throughout Europe between 1494 and 1498.[10,11,17] At this time, syphilis was a more acute disease and was frequently fatal during the second stage of infection.[11] It is believed that Columbus himself died of syphilis in 1506 from general paresis. Not until over 400 years later, in 1905, was the etiological agent, *Treponema pallidum*, discovered.[1,10,11,17] Syphilis was immediately recognized as being a new and previously unknown condition. In 1498, the first book on syphilis was written by Francisco Lopez de Villalobos, who recognized the venereal mode of spread and described the skin manifestations and later complications of syphilis.[11]

One of the first and most widely utilized "cures" for syphilis was guaiacum, "the sacred wood." The patient drank water into which guaiacum had been pounded and boiled. The primary and secondary, but not the late, manifestations of syphilis appeared to be favorably affected by this early form of syphilis chemotherapy. Mercury for the treatment of syphilis was first introduced in 1497 by Francisco Lopez de Villalobos, who deduced the idea from a study of old Arabic literature.[11] Given in correct dosage, mercury helped some patients; however, too much mercury caused serious damage, and it is unlikely that many patients were cured utilizing this treatment.[11,33] It was essential to give mercury in small amounts over many years, as illustrated by the phrase, "Five minutes with Venus, and a lifetime with mercury."[11] Most people, unwilling to wait 20 years for a cure, consulted magicians, quacks, and drug sellers, who often provided large dosages of mercury and left town prior to the appearance of mercury's side-effects: gum edema, ulcers of the mouth, and death from mercury poisoning.[11,33]

Progress in syphilis research was steady, if not spectacular, for several hundred years. Men such as Valambert, Fournier, Clutton, Diday, and Hutchinson made great contributions to the knowledge of syphilis by describing its clinical manifestations during its four stages.[10,11] Around 1530, Theophrastus Paracelsus became the first person of medical stature to hypothesize that gonorrhea and syphilis were different stages of the same disease. This debate continued until the self-experimentation of John

Hunter in 1767. Hunter obtained pus from a patient with gonorrhea and inoculated himself; unfortunately, the chosen patient also had syphilis, and despite treatment with mercury, Hunter developed cardiovascular syphilis and died in 1793. Hunter published his conclusion that gonorrhea and syphilis were the same disease in 1787; in 1838, however, Philippe Ricord demonstrated conclusively that the two were distinct diseases based upon his study of over 2,500 human inoculations.[11]

The period between 1905 and 1910 yielded three major discoveries that brought syphilis into the realm of medical management. In 1905, Fritz Schaudinn and Erich Hoffman saw and identified for the first time the spirochete *Treponema pallidum*, which causes syphilis.[11] In 1907, August von Wassermann and his associates developed the first blood test for the detection of syphilis. They worked on over 200 blood tests subsequent to their discovery; to this day, the search for sensitive and specific tests continues.[1,9,11] Also in 1907, Paul Ehrlich discovered an arsenic compound for the treatment of syphilis. It was his six hundred-sixth preparation, known as "Number 606, Salvarsan." It looked promising but was put aside by an assistant as it had not proven to be effective in animal experiments. In 1909, Sacachiro Hata repeated the experiments and proved that 606 was highly effective; in 1910, Ehrlich presented Salvarsan to the medical world as the first effective treatment against syphilis.[11]

In 1943, Dr. John Mahoney of the United States Public Health Service found that penicillin, discovered by Alexander Fleming in 1928, produced dramatic cures.[11] Penicillin, said to be a "wonder drug," quickly became the treatment of choice throughout the world..[1,11]

The problem today is not one of treating the patient but finding the patient who needs to be treated for syphilis. Our traditional attitude toward sexually transmitted diseases does little to encourage patients with such diseases to come forth for diagnosis and treatment.[1,10,11] Syphilis will probably remain epidemic until public attitudes change from moral condemnation to concern for the elimination of a major disease threat.[11]

Occurrence

Syphilis is presently the third most common reported communicable disease in the United States today, with approximately 22,000 cases reported and an actual estimated case load of 50,000 to 80,000 cases.[13,30,31] Approximately every 14 seconds, someone within the United States contracts either syphilis or gonorrhea.[13] It is presently estimated that some 510,000 people within the United States have syphilis and have not as yet been diagnosed and treated for it. Approximately 10,000 people are currently hospitalized for syphilitic psychoses; the direct cost of maintenance of these patients is estimated to be approximately $41 million per year.[45] Syphilis primarily involves young people between the ages of 15 and 30 years.[6] The disease is more prevalent in urban than rural areas and more frequent in males than females.[6]

Infectious Etiological Agent

Belonging to the order Spirochaetales and the family Treponemataceae, *Treponema pallidum* represents the etiological agent for venereal syphilis.[2,10] It varies from 5 to 15 microns in length and is of uniform cylindrical thickness of approximately .25 microns.[46] The organism generally exhibits 6 to 14 spirals and is actively motile, with motion produced by a corkscrew rotation rather than by flagella (hence the organism is not a true bacterium).[10,46] Motion as visualized by darkfield microscopy tends to be slowly backward and forward.[1,8,10,33] The typical method of division is by binary transverse fission, although some authorities claim that longitudinal division may also occur.[10,46] Spirochetes in general have cell walls which are rather membranous and flexible and are difficult to stain. To date, *Treponema pallidum* has not been successfully cultivated on artificial laboratory media, nor does it grow in embryonated chick eggs or in tissue cultures. The organism must be diagnosed upon the basis of microscopic characteristics, in material obtained from active lesions, or by serologic testing of the patient's serum.[8] While mankind is the natural host of *Treponema pallidum*, animals can be infected with this pathogenic microorganism experimentally.[1] It is important to note that there are several kinds of nonpathogenic treponema on the skin and within the mouth and vagina of healthy human beings.[10]

Reservoir and Source of Infection

Mankind is the only reservoir for venereal syphilis.[1,10] The source of infection is exudates (discharges) from obvious or concealed moist early lesions of the skin and mucous membranes of infected persons as well as body fluids and secretions (saliva, seminal fluid, blood, and vaginal discharges) during the infectious period (the primary and secondary stages of the disease).[1,6,10] Asymptomatic carriers of syphilis account for a large number of new infections, as approximately 40 to 60 percent of males and 90 percent of females do not recall a primary lesion (which tends to be painless and is often hidden or inconspicuous).[1,10,42]

Mode of Transmission

Transmission of syphilitic infection is by direct contact with an infected source, including sexual contact, kissing, and the fondling of children..[1,6,8] The infectious organism is not borne by food, water, air, or insects; there is no extrahuman reservoir of infection.[1,8,46] Stories of infection through contact with contaminated articles such as toilet seats, wet towels, chairs, drinking glasses, sheets, swimming pools, and domestic animals represent pure myth and deception. Despite all attempts, the organism has not been cultured away from living tissue.[46] It is readily killed by soap, ordinary antiseptics, drying, and heat.[8,10,33] It resists cold, however, and can be frozen or stored for long periods without loss of virulence.[33]

The spirochetes generally enter the body through intact mucous membranes but sometimes penetrate through breaks in the skin at the site of their deposit.[1,8] A condom does not provide definitive protection as the spirochetes may enter the skin above the condom or on the scrotum itself.[10,35,46] Once inside the body, *T. pallidum* is able to survive, despite body defenses, to become a systemic disease that may affect any organ.[42]

Some secretions, such as saliva and seminal fluid, are frequently in contact with infectious mucosal lesions and may contain *T. pallidum*. The blood of patients with early syphilis contains spirochetes and may not be utilized for transfusion purposes.[1,10,33,46] However, the serologic tests are not always an indication of the infectiousness of the blood, as syphilis can be transmitted by transfusion from patients in the incubation period or in the sero-negative primary stage of the disease.[33] The organism does not remain viable in whole blood or plasma which has been stored at refrigerator temperature for more than 96 hours.[33]

Incubation Period

Generally within 10 to 90 days (usually 3 to 4 weeks), a primary lesion or chancre appears at the portal of entry and persists for 1 to 5 weeks, healing spontaneously.[42,46] Approximately 6 weeks (2 weeks to 6 months) after the chancre disappears, the secondary manifestations of infection arise. Skin lesions of this stage will also heal spontaneously within 2 to 6 weeks. There follows a latency period of 2 to 50 years; then, finally, comes the onset of tertiary syphilis in approximately one-third of untreated patients.[1,10,42,46]

Period of Communicability or Infectivity

The period of communicability for venereal syphilis is variable and indefinite, but communicability is most common during the primary and secondary stages of disease and during periods of mucocutaneous recurrence. The World Health Organization has divided latent syphilis into early latent (duration under 4 years) and late latent (duration over 4 years); from an epidemiological standpoint, the WHO believes that only latent syphilis under one year's duration produces sufficient infectivity to warrant interviewing and contact investigation.[46] Every case of infectious syphilis must be considered the source for a potential epidemic, as no syphilitic case exists in isolation.[46] Definitive treatment generally ends infectivity within 24 hours.[6]

Susceptibility and Resistance

Susceptibility is universal with no natural immunity.[1,6] The natural resistance of mankind to virulent *T. pallidum* has been determined in volunteer subjects, in whom it was found that the ID_{50} for intracutaneous inoculation was approximately 57 organisms. Larger inoculations produced larger ulcerative lesions and shorter incubation periods.[33] However, virtually every patient with syphilis does develop some resistance to his own infection. (This resistance may be overcome by a large reinfecting dosage, or by eradication of the disease by treatment during the primary and secondary stages.[6,8]) The degree of immunity conferred determines whether the patient will achieve a spontaneous cure (approximately 25 percent of syphilitic patients), whether the disease will remain latent, or whether late complications will arise.[1,10,33] The factors responsible for the development of this particular type of immunity and the destruction of spirochetes are largely idiopathic.[33]

Epidemiology

Syphilitic epidemiology, while simple in theory, is difficult to apply because patients are often reluctant to name sexual contacts and physicians are reluctant to report cases, as opposed to simply treating them, due to time deficiencies.[46] The mobility of today's population demands prompt exchange of information to local potential asymptomatic infected contacts.[1,10,46] Contacts located but found not to be infected at first examination should be given prophylactic (preventive) treatment. Those known to have been exposed to "lesion or rash syphilis" should be given an STS and complete treatment; there is no point in waiting for the onset of clinical disease.[46]

Signs and Symptoms: Primary Syphilis

Following an incubation period of 10 to 90 days (average 21 days), a hard lesion or sore (chancre) appears at the portal of entry.[1,46] The surface of the primary lesion is crusted or ulcerated and there is an erythemic (red) border surrounded lesion in 50 percent of instances.[10] The lesion is not painful unless secondarily infected by bacteria, though extragenital chancres (sometimes found on the lips, tongue, tonsils, nipples, fingers, or anus) are more apt to cause pain.[1,10] They have a raw border which is raised and firm (like the edges of a button) and an indurated center. Generally, the chancre is "ham-colored," does not bleed easily, and is single; however, multiple lesions are not rare.[10,46] The size of the lesion may be from a few millimeters to 1 or 2 centimeters in diameter. It must be noted that the appearance of chancres can vary considerably, from a slight erosion to a deep ulcer; that is, no "typical" lesion exists, as there are many varieties of primary syphilitic lesions.[10,42]

Even without treatment, the chancre heals completely within 4 to 6 weeks; if the lesion has been present for 4 weeks or longer, nearly all reagin tests will be reactive.[1,46] Upon healing, the chancre may leave a mild scar not readily visible to the untrained eye.[10]

Inguinal lymphadenopathy (satellite bubo), representing enlarged, hard, and painless lymph nodes, is common in instances of primary and secondary syphilis.[1,10,46] A darkfield examination of fluid obtained through needle aspiration of a bubo can be diagnostic in instances where insufficient fluid is obtained from the chancre itself.[1,10,33,46] This diagnostic procedure is also helpful in instances where topical medications have been applied to the chancre or where the lesion is inconspicuous.[46]

In particular, careful examination is essential to the detection of chancres in women and in gay or bisexual males.[1,10,46] According to the Center for Disease Control in Atlanta, Georgia, all genital lesions should be assumed to be syphilitic until definitively proven otherwise.[9,12]

Signs and Symptoms: Secondary Syphilis

If primary syphilis remains untreated, the disease progresses into its secondary stage with the following clinical manifestations generally evident within approximately 6 weeks (2 weeks to 6 months) following the disappearance of the chancre:[1,6,8,10,17,46]

Generalized syphilitic dermatitis appears. This skin rash is highly variable in appearance and location upon the body; it is transient in nature even without treatment, and may be accompanied by constitutional symptoms.[1,10,44] The lesions are usually on the palms of the hands and the soles of the feet but may be generalized over the entire body.[23] Upon the face, the rash may form in "rings".[10] The rash does not itch and is not painful.[1,46] On white skin, the rash initially appears cherry- or ham-colored and then becomes a copper or brownish color as fading occurs, generally within a few weeks.[1,10] In black patients, the rash presents as a grayish-blue color.[10] The skin lesions are bilaterally symmetrical and may be macular, papular, follicular, papulosquamous, or pustular in nature; vesiculobullous lesions do not occur in adults, but may be seen in neonatal congenital syphilis.[46] These lesions represent foci of disseminated spirochetes and may occur at numerous sites such as skin, bones, joints, eyes, mucosa, and the central nervous system.[8] Like the primary chancre, superficial secondary lesions teem with spirochetes and are infectious.[8] As a rule, *Treponema pallidum* may be obtained from any mucous or cutaneous secondary lesion, but most easily from a moist one.[46] However, failure to demonstrate the organism in this matter does not rule out the diagnosis.[10,46] In secondary relapsing syphilis, the lesions tend to be arciform and may be asymmetrical.[46]

Alopecia or hair loss occurs. "Moth-eaten" scalp alopecia beginning in the occipital region is most characteristic; however, alopecia may occur anywhere on the scalp and may result in the loss of eyelashes and the lateral third of the eyebrows.[1,10,33,46] This hair will grow back following definitive treatment.

Moist papules or lesions occur most frequently in the anogenital region, mouth, and intertriginous surfaces.[46] Lesions of the mouth, throat, and cervix may sometimes occur while the primary chancre is still present and are characteristic of secondary syphilis.[1,10,46]

Generalized lymphadenopathy and splenomegaly are characteristic of secondary syphilis.[1,10,46]

Constitutional symptoms occur in approximately 25 percent of syphilitic patients, who experience a generalized feeling of "ill health" characterized by headache, fever, pharyngitis, anorexia, constipation, and pain within long bones, muscles, and joints.[10]

As with the chancre, secondary syphilitic symptomology becomes asymptomatic even without treatment in approximately 2 to 6 weeks (sometimes longer) of their appearance.[1,10,33] Rarely, systemic manifestations of hepatitis, iritis, nephritis, osteomyelitis, and meningitis may be seen.[42]

Atypical manifestations of secondary syphilis occasionally appear. In pregnant women, primary chancres of the vaginal lips may be prominent, while the secondary rash may be highly inconspicuous.[10,33] Exclusively in black patients, an annular, hyperpigmented lesion of the face, almost pathognomonic, with a raised border is sometimes seen.[42] As the clinical manifestations of primary and secondary syphilis vary so greatly, suspicion should be aroused by any localized or generalized nonpruritic symmetrical eruption accompanied by generalized or inguinal lymphadenopathy and confirmed by laboratory tests.[1,10,33,42]

Signs and Symptoms: Latent Syphilis

The secondary syphilitic eruption heals within 2 to 8 weeks without scarring, and other signs and symptoms disappear, heralding the beginning of latent syphilis.[42] This third stage of syphilis thus generally begins from 6 months to 2 years after the initial infection; it may last for years.[1,10,17] The disease is termed *early latent syphilis* when it has been present for less than 4 years or if the patient is under 25 years of age;

infections persisting for more than 4 years or involving patients over 25 years of age are termed *late latent infections*.[17] The latent period is dangerously deceptive because symptomology is absent. It was during this stage of disease in the great syphilitic epidemic of the fifteenth century that the condition was thought to be cured.[17] In approximately 25 percent of latent syphilis patients, the secondary rash tends to recur along with other potential secondary signs and symptoms periodically for approximately 2 years after infection; in some instances this relapse of secondary syphilitic symptomology continues for even longer periods.[1,10,42] After 4 years of infection, relapsing infectious lesions are very rare. Latency may be lifelong, or late syphilis may appear within 2 years of the initial infection.[1,10,46] It should be noted that all syphilis is latent at some time during its clinical course.

The diagnosis of latent syphilis is based upon a reactive, repeatable blood serology without other laboratory or clinical findings; a treponemal test such as the FTA-ABS will substantiate or refute the diagnosis.[1,33] A clinical diagnosis of latent syphilis does not preclude entirely the potential for infectiousness or the development of gummatous lesions, cardiovascular abnormalities, and/or neurosyphilis; should such become apparent, the diagnosis then is no longer latent, but tertiary or late syphilis.[1,46]

Tertiary or Late Syphilis

Late syphilis, the fourth stage of the disease, may manifest itself in any organ of the body as late as 30 to 50 years following the initial infection.[1,17,46] The estimate is that approximately 20 to 50 percent of those exposed to syphilis contract the disease (depending upon whether the infection is primary or secondary) and that of those who remain untreated, one-third will develop late syphilis, specifically in the forms of late benign syphilis (17 percent), cardiovascular syphilis (10 percent), and neurosyphilitic diseases (8 percent).[1,10,17,46] These divisions are not mutually exclusive: 13 percent of patients with late benign syphilis have cardiovascular involvement and another 10 percent neurosyphilis;[46] of patients with cardiovascular syphilis, approximately 12 percent have associated neurosyphilis; and of all patients with neurosyphilis, approximately 15 percent have associated cardiovascular syphilis.[46]

The mortality rate for all patients with untreated syphilis is approximately 23 percent. Cardiovascular complications are responsible for approximately 80 percent of deaths, with most of the remaining deaths arising from central nervous system (brain and spinal cord) involvement.[1,46]

Those untreated patients who do not develop late syphilis (approximately two-thirds) live their lives with minimal or no complications, although more than 50 percent will remain serologically positive for life.[1,10,46] Unfortunately, there is no means of predicting which patients will develop the clinical manifestations of late syphilis and which ones will not.[1,10,46]

Tertiary Benign Syphilis or Late Benign Syphilis

Today, late syphilis is extremely rare in the United States; the most common form is late benign syphilis, accounting for 17 percent of reported cases. The manifestations of late benign syphilis generally appear within 3 to 7 years after infection. The medical term "benign" denotes that the gummas or destructive ulcers characteristic of this form of syphilis rarely result in total physical incapacity or death.[46]

It must be remembered that, from beginning to end, syphilis is essentially a vascular disease, with the exception of gummas, which are probably a hypersensitivity reaction. Aside from gummas, late syphilitic lesions are produced by obliterative endarteritis of the terminal arterioles (small arteries) and by the consequent inflammatory and necrotic changes produced.[46]

Tertiary benign syphilis may affect the skin, muscles, digestive organs, liver, lungs, eyes, and endocrine organs.[1,33] Characteristically, the gumma develops on or in the affected organ. If treated promptly, the gumma heals, with the patient recovering completely in most instances.[10] (Technically, when such gummas or late destructive ulcers arise in the brain or other vital organs, the term "benign" is misleading and inaccurate.)[46] The skin lesions may be solitary or multiple, tend to form in a circular pattern or in segments of circles, and are destructive and chronic in nature.[10,33] Symptoms of syphilitic bone infections include gummatous osteitis with bone destruction, pain, edema (swelling), and a bony neoplasm (tumor) which most commonly affects the skull, tibia, and/or clavicle.[10,24] In late benign syphilis, the STS are almost always reactive and generally of a high titer.[10]

Tertiary Cardiovascular Syphilis or Cardiovascular Late Syphilis

The second most common form of tertiary or late syphilis is cardiovascular syphilis, which affects 10 percent of all untreated patients after 10 to 40 years of untreated syphilitic infection.[10] The infection produces injury to the heart and major blood vessels, often resulting in death. Specifically, lesions are caused by medial necrosis of the aorta, with aortic dilatation often extending into the aortic valve commissures.[46] Principal signs include aortic insufficiency, saccular aneurysm (weakening) of the thoracic aorta, and a history of hypertension, arteriosclerosis (hardening of the arteries), and previous rheumatic cardiovascular disease.[10] Aortic insufficiency with no other valvular lesions in a middle-aged person with reactive STS should be considered cardiovascular syphilis until proven otherwise.[10] The STS in patients with cardiovascular syphilis are generally reactive.[46]

Tertiary Neurosyphilis

Approximately 8 percent of all untreated patients with syphilitic infections develop one or more forms of neurosyphilis within 10 to 20 years of infection.[10,33] This infection affects the central nervous system (brain and spinal cord), producing paralysis and/or paresis (insanity).[1,10,24,33] *Clinical Symposia on Syphilis*, developed by CIBA Pharmaceutical Company, details the potential manifestations of neurosyphilis in excellent fashion as follows:[46]

1. **Asymptomatic neurosyphilis** — The patient is generally seen due to reactive STS with no symptoms of CNS involvement. Examination of the spinal fluid is abnormal, with an increase in cells, total protein, and a reactive VDRL or Kolmer compliment fixation text.

2. **Meningovascular neurosyphilis** — Definite symptomology of CNS damage exists resulting from cerebrovascular occlusion, infarction, and encephalomalacia, with spinal fluid always abnormal.

3. **Parenchymatous neurosyphilis** presents as either *paresis* or *tabes dorsalis*. In paresis, personality changes may range from minor to psychotic, with focal neurological signs frequent, abnormal cerebrospinal fluid (cells and proteins increased), and a VDRL and compliment fixation test which are both reactive. Typical manifestations of tabes dorsalis include posterior column degeneration, ataxia, areflexia, paresthesias, bladder disturbances, impotency, and lancinating pain. Trophic joint changes (*Charcot's joints*) result from loss or impairment of the sensation of pain, with the knee joint most commonly affected. Loss of deep pain sensation may be associated with perforating ulcers on the soles or toes (*Mal perforans*). Optic atrophy is a serious complication of neurosyphilis. Pupil changes most commonly seen include the Argyll-Robertson pupil, which is small, irregular, and fails to respond to light (but does respond to normal convergence). The cerebrospinal fluid (CSF) is abnormal in approximately 90 percent of instances, and STS are reactive in some 75 percent of patients.

It is important to note that all neurosyphilis is asymptomatic at some time during its clinical course and that it is rare for neurosyphilis to present in a "pure" form.[46] In all forms, the essential pathophysiology is the same: obliterative endarteritis, generally of terminal vessels, with associated parenchymateous degeneration, which may or may not be sufficient at the time of examination to produce symptoms.[1,10,33,46]

Syphilis During Pregnancy

During pregnancy, primary syphilitic chancres upon the vaginal lips may be more prominent than usual; however, other symptomology, such as the secondary syphilitic rash, may be absent or highly inconscipuous.[10] Following the eighteenth week of pregnancy, when the Langhans' cell layer of the early placenta has atrophied, the spirochetes may cross the placental barrier to infect the fetus.[46] Pregnancy during a mother's primary or secondary infection results in miscarriage, stillbirth, or congenital infection of the fetus in 90 percent of instances.[44] Pregnancy in the later stages of syphilis may result in a clinical spectrum from a fulminating fatal congenital syphilis to an uninfected child.[46] Thus, the more recent the infection in the mother, the more likely the infant is to be infected and the more likely the complications are to be serious.[1,10,33,46] The vast majority of congenital infections are acquired with 4 years of maternal infection; however, the disease can apparently be transmitted to the fetus for 10 years or more after the onset of disease.

Adequate treatment of the mother prior to the eighteenth week of pregnancy prevents infection of the fetus. As penicillin crosses the placental barrier, treatment of the mother after the eighteenth week will also cure the fetus.[1,10,33,46] A woman who is given definitive treatment and followed with quantitative STS, and with no evidence of reinfection, does not need to be treated with each subsequent pregnancy.[46] However, when any doubt exists concerning the adequacy of previous treatment or the presence of an active infection, a full course of treatment should be given to cure the mother and prevent congenital syphilis.[1,10,46] Of academic interest is the finding that pregnancy appears to have a beneficial influence upon the course of syphilitic infection in the mother, with late manifestations of the disease less frequent in multiparous women than in others.[33] Studies reveal that maternal syphilitic infection becomes more attenuated as the duration of the disease increases, with the chances for fetal infection diminished with each succeeding pregnancy.[23,33]

A serologic test for syphilis (STS) should be taken at the first prenatal visit of every pregnant woman (preferably before the fourth month); a second STS should be performed during the sixth month, and a third test during the ninth month.[1,10,33] The early recognition of syphilis in pregnancy followed by definitive treatment prevents congenital syphilis in virtually every instance.[33]

Congenital Syphilis

Congenital syphilis is divided into two categories: early and late.[1,8,24] Since *Treponema pallidum* is introduced directly into the fetal circulation, there is no primary stage.[1,33,46]

Syphilitic disease that presents clinically before age 2 is categorized as "early."[1,33] Dermatologic lesions of early congenital syphilis are similar to those of secondary syphilis; however, involvement of major organs such as the lungs, pancreas, meninges, and bone make this infection even more severe and life-threatening.[1,33] Neonates with overt congenital syphilis characteristically present with marasmus, snuffles, pot belly, "old man" faces, mucocutaneous lesions, and pseudoparalysis; however, the majority are born asymptomatic and do not develop signs or symptoms until the third or fourth week. In some, the only manifestation may be a reactive STS.[1,33] Other signs are as follows:

1. Cutaneous lesions appear shortly after birth. The skin lesions are at first frequently vesicular or bullous, progressing to superficial crusted lesions. Developing later, the lesions are papulosquamous, with a generalized symmetrical distribution similar to acquired syphilis; they may form typical condylomata lata.

2. Mucous-membrane lesions are present, often involving the nasopharynx, producing a heavy mucoid exudate referred to as "snuffles." Hemmorrhagic nasal exudate in the neonate is characteristic of syphilis. Both skin and mucous membrane lesions teem with spirochetes, rendering such lesions and exudates extremely infectious. A positive diagnosis can be established by darkfield examination.

3. Bone abnormalities. — While only 15 percent of infants evidence clinical signs, virtually 100 percent will show radiologic evidence of osteochondritis of the long bones following the first month of life. Dactylitis results from involvement of the phalanges.

4. A self-limited, hemolytic anemia is common.

5. Hepatosplenomegaly will be found in two-thirds of patients. This sign may be associated with a low-grade icterus.

6. Central nervous system involvement. — Up to one half of infants may have abnormal spinal fluid, although the incidence of clinical manifestations is much lower.

Late congenital syphilis presents clinically after 2 years of age.[1] In 60 percent of cases, the disease is latent, with no clinical manifestations other than reactive STS.[10,46] The disease processes associated with late congenital syphilis are potentially as follows:[46]

1. Interstitial keratitis. — Near puberty, the cornea develops a ground-glass appearance; the condition becomes bilateral and leads to blindness.

2. Hutchinson's teeth. — The permanent upper incisors develop a barrel-shaped notched appearance. Diagnosis is by x-ray examination.

3. Mulberry or Moon's molars. — The first molars may show maldevelopment of the cusps.

4. Eighth nerve deafness, while not common, sometimes occurs at puberty or even into middle age.

5. Neurosyphilis. — Clinical course as for acquired syphilis.

6. Bone Abnormality. — Perforation of the hard palate.

7. Cutaneous lesions (rhagades) arising from infantile syphilitic rhinitis are rarely seen. Gummas may involve the skin or other organs.

8. Cardiovascular lesions are relatively rare but have been seen.

9. Clutton's joints. — A painless hydrarthrosis, generally of the knees and rarely involving the elbows or other large joints may occur.

Interstitial keratitis, eighth nerve deafness, and Clutton's joints are often associated with each other near puberty. This triad does not respond well to penicillin and is thought to be a hypersensitivity phenomenon rather than a purely spirochetal involvement of the structures.[46]

Undetected congenital syphilis generally manifests itself early in life, but symptoms may not appear until 30 years of age or later.[1,10,17,33] Pupillary abnormalities or varying degrees of mental defect, ranging from mild to severe, as well as cerebral developmental defects are among the more common signs presented.[17]

Doctors McCary and McCary, authors of *McCary's Human Sexuality*, have noted that congenital syphilis has greatly diminished within recent years due to improved routine prenatal care and treatment of pregnant women.[17] In 1941, there were 13,600 reported cases of congenital syphilis diagnosed in children under one year of age; by 1970, that figure had dropped to 300 cases.[17] Studies by Pund and others have shown that, indeed, a syphilitic mother generally transmits the disease to any child she conceives during the first 2 years of her infection; treated prior to the fourth month of pregnancy, only 1 in 11 infants is born with congenital syphilis.[17]

Diagnosis of Venereal Syphilis

The diagnosis of syphilis is not easy; the disease can produce symptomology quite similar to a variety of other diseases, such as psoriasis, cancer, infectious mononucleosis, drug reactions, etc.[1,10,33] Many variables must be given thorough consideration, such as the patient's complete personal and family medical history; the presence or absence of syphilis and/or other forms of STD in the patient's sexual partner(s); the clinical manifestations of disease presented by the patient; and the results of laboratory tests to detect syphilis and other potentially present forms of STD.

It must be clearly understood that venereal syphilis is a systemic disease affecting all parts of the patient's body.[1,10] The examining physician should carefully inspect the patient's genital region, rectum, pharynx, entire skin surface, eyes, lungs, and abdomen. Vital signs, including pulse, blood pressure, respiratory rate and function, and temperature, should be carefully assessed on all patients.[1,33] Any allergies or medications which the patient is presently taking should be noted in particular. Should a chancre be present, nothing should be applied topically; while almost any chemical substance applied will kill spirochetes upon the skin's surface, systemic disease will continue, and diagnosis will be made more difficult by subsequent distorted microscopic morphology of *T. pallidum*.[1,10]

General Diagnostic Approach for Patients with Potential STD

Every patient should have an RPR (Rapid Plasma Reagin) test and complete cultures for gonorrhea. Diagnostic techniques for gonorrhea may be found on pages 28-32 (men) and 32-35 (women); laboratory techniques may be found on pages 35-39.

Laboratory Diagnosis

To establish a definitive diagnosis of venereal syphilis, laboratory tests are necessary.[1,10,42] Darkfield examination is most useful in the early stages of syphilis and should be utilized in conjunction with serologic tests when possible to establish the diagnosis.[1,33]

1. The darkfield examination. — Because *T. pallidum* is not readily stained by ordinary laboratory methods and is so similar to other spirochetes inhabiting the oral cavity and genitalia of healthy individuals, it is essential whenever possible to examine the organism in its living state.[8,46] Darkfield examination represents the direct microscopic examination of serous material obtained from a moist lesion of primary or secondary syphilis or from a dry indurated lesion whose surface can be eroded and from which serum can be obtained.[1,42] The darkfield microscope is designed to block out the central rays of light and to direct the peripheral rays across the field so that the organism is seen by reflected light.[33,42] Particles in suspension are brightly illuminated (and may appear larger due to the reflected light, which spreads outward in a cone); the background is very dark as only light that is reflected from particle surfaces can enter the lens.[8] When spirochetes are visualized in this manner, they are seen distinctly, gleaming with light in the dark field. Other particles in the preparation also shine, but treponemes can be readily distinguished from other organisms present in the exudate by their characteristic motility and morphology.[1,6,8,10,33,46]

Certain precautions must be taken in order to obtain a satisfactory specimen. In collecting specimens for examination, plastic or rubber gloves should be worn to protect the examiner from accidental infection.[46] The surface of a lesion must be cleaned of superficial debris and rubbed somewhat vigorously with a cotton sponge and saline to obtain free-flowing serum from the base of the lesion.[42,46] The lesion is then dried and gently abraded to the point of bleeding.[10,46] When clear serum exudes, a drop is picked up directly upon the surface of a glass slide and a cover slip is placed over it. Should there be much delay before examination, the edges of the cover slip must be covered with petroleum jelly.[46]

Darkfield examination must be performed by an experienced person, as there are other spirochetes in the oral and genital region which can be easily confused with *T. pallidum*.[1,8,42] Oral lesions are often misinterpreted, as *Treponema microdentium*, a common saprophytic resident of the mouth, very closely simulates the morphology of *T. pallidum*.[8,10,24,42] If the patient has utilized topical antibiotics or antiseptics for the lesion or if the lesion is secondarily contaminated, the organism may be temporarily destroyed in the surface serum.[42] Under such circumstances, the patient should be advised to soak the lesion in saline solution 3 or 4 times per day and return 24 hours later for repeated darkfield examination.[10,42] When the lesion is inaccessible, such as under a tight foreskin, lymph node puncture will reveal the organism.[42] Under proper circumstances and with appropriate precautions, the darkfield examination is accurate and permits an immediate diagnosis of early syphilis.[33,42]

2. Serological tests.—The darkfield examination is limited to "lesion" cases; it is estimated that approximately 70 percent of venereal syphilis is diagnosed on the basis of blood tests, as 40 to 60 percent of males and 90 percent of females do not recall the presence of a chancre.[1,10,42]

There are two groups of blood tests which measure serologic (antibody) response to syphilitic infections: *reagin* and *treponemal*. The reagin tests measure antibodies to a nonspecific antigen (beef-heart extract fortified with cholesterol and lecithin). The most widely utilized prototype tests are the RPR and the VDRL (Rapid Plasma Reagin and Venereal Disease Research Laboratory, respectively).[10,42,46] The treponemal tests have as the antigen the organism itself, the prototype being the FTA-ABS, or Fluorescent Treponemal Antibody Absorption Test.[42,46]

A. Nontreponemal antigen (reagin) tests. While these tests are not absolutely specific or sensitive for syphilis, their performance is quite practical, and they are widely utilized, with their findings undoubtedly indicative of possible infection.[8,42] Although some people still utilize the term "Wassermann" for any nontreponemal STS, that test is no longer performed, and the term should be dropped.[46]

Reagin is generally first detected in the serum approximately 4 to 6 weeks after infection or 1 to 3 weeks after the chancre appears.[8,10,42] A rising titer may indicate a recent infection, reinfection in an adequately treated patient, relapse of an inadequately treated patient, or an acute false-positive reaction.[33,46] Adequate treatment of early syphilitic infection is indicated by a decline in the patient's titer.[8,24,42]

Careful attention should be paid to every reactive or weakly reactive STS. Some of the highest titers recorded have been in patients with late visceral or cutaneous syphilis or in nonsyphilitic diseases such as hemolytic anemia or systemic lupus erythematosus.[10,46]

Titers generally become nonreactive in approximately 6 to 12 months following the treatment of primary syphilis and in 12 to 18 months following chemotherapy for secondary syphilis.[1,33,46] Treatment upon a late or latent infection generally has little or no effect upon the titer and should not be utilized to gauge the adequacy of chemotherapy.[1,10,33,46]

(1) *The Venereal Disease Research Laboratory (VDRL) test is utilized to establish a more definitive diagnosis in instances where a darkfield examination has been positive.*[10] The test is relatively inexpensive, accurate, and easy to perform; however, it cannot provide accurate results prior to 7-10 days after the primary lesion appears.[10,42] In very early cases of syphilis or in some late stages of the disease, the test may be nonreactive even though syphiltic infection exists; the test provides a false negative in 24 percent of primary syphilitic cases. False positives may be obtained with recent infections of measles, chickenpox, mononucleosis, infectious hepatitis, recent smallpox vaccinations, rat-bite fever, and in pregnant women.[1,10,33] Long-lasting false positives may occur in people with systemic lupus erythematosus, rheumatoid arthritis, drug addicts (60 percent of positives are false), chancroid, lymphogranuloma venereum, dysproteinemia, and Hashimoto's thyroiditis.[1,10,33]

(2) *The Rapid Plasma Reagin (RPR) test* is utilized for the rapid screening of sera. The RPR involves the utilization of a modified VDRL antigen, and the test is made more sensitive by the addition of choline chloride.[8,46] Blood is collected in anticoagulant tubes, centrifuged, and tested immediately, without heating the plasma.[1,46] The RPR antigen has been adapted to perform a similar test on the plasma portion of a microhematocrit determination (Plasmacrit or PCT test).[46] After reading the packed-cell volume, the capillary tube is divided, and the plasma expressed for testing.[8,42] The PCT test has been particularly useful in blood bank operations to exclude donors before collection, in screening hospital admissions, and as capillary specimens are utilized, in testing infants.[46]

B. The Fluorescent Treponemal Antibody Absorption Test (FTA-

ABS. The FTA blood tests are the most recent and promising tests developed to date. The best of these is the FTA-ABS.[46] Although more expensive and difficult to perform, as only fairly recently has the test been completely automated, its specificity and sensitivity make the FTA-ABS today the confirmatory test of choice.[1,8,10,34,46] The test is 99 percent specific and is more sensitive than the other blood tests in all stages of venereal syphilis.[10] False positives are much less common, and the test becomes reactive earlier in early syphilis than does the RPR, VDRL, and formerly utilized TPI.[46] However, as previously stated, a number of diseases may produce a false positive serology. Repeatedly reactive STS accompanied by nonreactive FTA-ABS characterize a false-positive reactor.[33,46] The duration of reagin activity arbitrarily determines whether the false-positive reaction is acute (less than 6 months) or chronic (more than 6 months).[33,46]

C. Spinal Fluid Examination. A sample of the cerebrospinal fluid surrounding the spinal column is taken by needle aspiration through the vertebra. Three tests are then utilized to diagnose potential neurosyphilis:[46]

(1) *Cell count* — The presence of more than 4 lymphocytes is considered abnormal.[10,46]

(2) *Total protein* — The protein fraction is always elevated in instances of active neurosyphilis.

(3) *Kolmer or VDRL spinal fluid tests* — Examination for the presence of reagin within the spinal fluid; false-positives in spinal fluid examination are exceedingly rare.[10,46]

Spinal fluid examination represents the only means of accurately diagnosing neurosyphilis and evaluating its treatment.[46] Not infrequently, neurosyphilis can be demonstrated months or years before the development of subjective and objective neurological evidence of the disease.[33,46] In the early forms of syphilis, CSF study is most meaningful 6 months to a year posttreatment[46], while in latent and late syphilis, examination should precede treatment.[1,33,46] A diagnosis of latent syphilis cannot be made unless asymptomatic neurosyphilis is excluded by a negative CSF examination.[46]

*Differential Diagnosis of Syphilis: Primary Stage**

Any genital lesion must be considered suspect of primary syphilis until ruled out by clinical and laboratory diagnosis.[46]

1. Chancroid. These lesions are generally multiple, soft, tender erosions or ulcerations with a grayish base. Both the lesions and associated lymphadenopathy are often more pronounced upon one side, and are quite

---

*From *Clinical Symposia on Syphilis*, CIBA Pharmaceutical Co., Summit, N.J. 07901

painful. While darkfield examination is negative, *H. ducreyi* may be demonstrated from the lesion by direct stained smear or by culture. Occasionally, a false-positive, low-titered STS may be noted.

2. Granuloma inguinale. — This disease is characterized by a soft, painless, raised, raw beef-colored, smooth, granulating lesion. Darkfield and STS are negative, and no significant lymphadenopathy occurs. The pathognomonic Donovan bodies, formerly *Donovanian granulomatis*, now *Calymmatobacterium granulomatis*, are best demonstrated by direct-tissue-spread smears stained with such dyes as Wright's stain. Biopsy may demonstrate the causative organisms and rule out carcinoma.

3. Lymphogranuloma venereum (LGV). — The initial lesion is a small, transient, rarely seen vesiculo-ulcer. The patient generally shows unilateral, painful inguinale lymphadenopathy. *T. pallidum, C. granulomatis*, and *H. ducreyi* should be excluded by specific studies. A rising titer detected by complement-fixation tests against the causative organism (*Chlamydial lymphogranulomatis*) is diagnostic.

4. Herpes progenitalis. — This viral process is generally manifested by grouped, painful, vesicular lesions. The history usually reveals recurrent lesions at the same site. A smear will demonstrate typical "balloon" cells. This virus is easily isolated directly from lesions where this laboratory service is available.

5. Carcinoma. — Generally the lesion has been present for a considerable period of time; the definitive diagnosis is by biopsy.

6. Scabies. — Pruritic vesicles with burrow formation are highly suggestive, and finding the mite in the burrow is diagnostic. The burrow may provide a break in the skin for inoculation of *T. pallidum*.

7. Lichen planus. — Genital lesions are generally annular or the typical polygonal, flat-topped, violaceous papules. They may be pruritic and may be single or multiple. The STS are nonreactive.

8. Psoriasis. — This disease often presents an erythematous or erythematosquamous plaque on the glans. Removal of the scale produces pinpoint bleeding; STS are nonreactive.

9. Drug eruptions. — The genital region is a frequent site of "fixed" dermatitis medicamentosa. Antipyrine, phenolphthalein, phenacetin, barbiturates, salicylates, sulfonamides, and antibiotics are among the most common offenders. The STS are generally nonreactive.

10. Aphthosis. — Along with oral and ocular lesions, aphthosis appears as round to polycyclic, painful, mucous-membrane erosions upon the genitalia.

11. Deep mycotic infections. — Deep fungi may produce chancriform genital lesions. The diagnosis is based upon potassium hydroxide preparations, culture, and biopsy. The STS are nonreactive.

12. Reiter's syndrome. — Nonspecific urethritis, conjunctivitis, and polyarthritis constitute the syndrome; superficial lesions of the glans may occur.

Differential Diagnosis of Venereal Syphilis: Secondary Stage*

1. Pityriasis rosea. — Erythematous, maculopapulosquamous lesions occur along the lines of skin cleavage, generally sparing the distal parts of the extremities, head, and neck, as well as mucous membranes. The body eruption is often preceded for one or more weeks by a single lesion, the herald patch. Darkfield examination is negative and the STS nonreactive.

2. Psoriasis. — Erythematous, maculopapulosquamous lesions commonly appear on the scalp, elbows, knees, chest, back, and buttocks. The nails and intertriginous regions may be involved. Pinpoint bleeding results from manual removal of scales. A history of chronicity is generally obtained. The darkfield examination is negative, the STS nonreactive.

3. Lichen planus. — Violaceous, papular, pruritic lesions occur most commonly upon the wrists, ankles, and sacral regions. Genital and oral lesions may occur. The darkfield examination is negative and STS nonreactive.

4. Tinea versicolor. — Brown, superficial, scaly lesions, which may be erythematous, are typical. Scrapings for spores and hyphae are positive.

5. "Id" eruptions. — Lesions are diversified, but may be papulosquamous, macular, or vesicular. Dermatophyte infection, bacterial infection, and/or eczematous processes can generally be found in other parts of the body. The darkfield examination is negative; STS are nonreactive.

6. Perleche. — The fissured split papules occurring at the angles of the mouth in secondary syphilis mimic the fissuring occasionally associated with cheilitis, hypovitaminosis, and oral moniliasis. The STS are negative.

7. Parasites. — Scabies and pediculosis infestations are suggested by

---

*From *Clinical Symposia on Syphilis*, CIBA Pharmaceutical Co., Summit, N.J. 07901.

excoriated papules and pustules often found in intertriginous regions. Pruritus is severe. Demonstration of the parasite is diagnostic.

8. Iritis and neuroretinitis. — When these conditions are part of the secondary syphilis syndrome, they are accompanied by other recognizable lesions. The STS will be *reactive*.

9. Condylomata acuminata. — These verrucous acuminate lesions, which are of viral etiology, are most frequently seen around the glans, vulva, and rectal regions. Darkfield examination may reveal large numbers of saprophytic treponemes, but no *T. pallidum*. The STS are nonreactive.

10. Acute exanthemata. — Epidemic, generalized, morbilliform, occasionally petechial eruptions associated with fever and other constitutional symptoms are the usual manifestations. The darkfield examination is negative and the STS generally nonreactive.

11. Infectious mononucleosis. — The generalized eruption (present in approximately 10 percent of patients), lymphadenopathy, and inflamed pharynx closely resemble secondary syphilis. *Very rarely*, some of the STS are *reactive*, and the spleen may be markedly enlarged. Careful darkfield examination of lesions may be essential to exclude syphilis. Atypical lymphocytes in the blood smear and a positive heterophile agglutination test establish the diagnosis.

12. Alopecia. — The nonscarring, temporary hair loss of secondary syphilis is generally associated with other characteristic cutaneous lesions. STS are uniformly reactive, and the darkfield examination of moist lesions occurring elsewhere will be positive for *T. pallidum*. Toxic and traumatic alopecia, as well as alopecia areata, may be ruled out by history, examination of the hair, negative darkfield examination, and nonreactive STS.

It must be noted and emphasized that any of the differential conditions may occur concurrently with venereal syphilis.[1,33,46]

Summary Statement on Differential Diagnosis

In differential diagnosis, venereal syphilis may be ruled out by the following factors:[46]

1. Darkfield examination studies. — Combined with:

2. Serologic reagin tests. — Both qualitative and quantitative, and:

3. Specific Treponemal tests. — Particularly the FTA-ABS if the above are equivocal; however, it must be remembered that:

A. Many nonvenereal genital diseases mimic primary syphilitic infections.

B. Extragenital chancres are *not* uncommon.

C. Other forms of STD or nonvenereal disease may coexist with primary or any other stage of syphilitic infection.

4. Careful history and physical examination. — An accurate history is essential to the diagnosis and treatment of syphilis or other conditions which mimic it. The physician should speak the language of the layman, and the routine medical history should include the following:

A. The chief complaint (CC).
B. The history of past and present illness.
C. Social history.
D. System review.

Specifically, the routine medical history should include:[46]

A. Remembered symptomology (prior lesions of the skin or genitalia, eye complaints, hair loss, etc.).

B. Parental or family infections (blood tests, stillbirths, etc.).

C. Previous STS — (premarital, employment, hospitalization) and lumbar puncture.

D. Treatment — Which might include antiluetic (hip and arm shots).

The necessity of a careful and complete physical examination, including neurological evaluation and a routine STS, cannot be overstressed. The patient should be completely unclothed, and all cutaneous surfaces, including the mucous membranes and anogenital region, inspected in good light, preferably daylight.[46]

*Specific Diagnosis and Recommended Chemotherapy**

1. Primary veneral syphilis

A. Symptomology. — A hard, indurated chancre which is generally painless and is usually confined to the genital region but may appear elsewhere. The chancre has an erythic (red) border in 50 percent of instances and heals even without treatment in 4 to 6 weeks.[46] If secondarily infected, the chancre may be painful; often the chancre is inconspicuous (40 to 60 percent of males and 90 percent of females), particularly for females or gay or bisexual males.[10] There may be inguinal lymphadenopathy.

B. Diagnosis. — Darkfield examination of serous exudate from lesion; RPR or VDRL.*

C. Treatment. — Penicillin G. Benzathine 2.4 mu/IM times one.

From the Pennsylvania Department of Public Health, Division of Acute Infectious Diseases.

D. Alternative treatment.—Penicillin G procaine 600,000 u/IM q.i.d. for 8 days; Tetracycline hydrochloride (HCL) 500 mg p.o./q.i.d. for 15 days; Erythromycin 500 mg p.o./q.i.d. for 15 days.

2. **Secondary venereal syphilis**
   A. Symptomology.—Rash (any type of lesion except vesicular) particularly upon the palms and soles but may be anywhere on the body. Less obvious in pregnant women, the rash is generally cherry- or ham-colored and then fades. In black patients, the rash may appear grayish blue. It may form in ring patterns upon the face in all syphilitic patients. Headache, fever, sore throat, malaise, alopecia (hair loss) particularly in the occipital region along with loss of eyelashes and the lateral one-third of the eyebrows may occur.[1,10,33] Mucous membrane lesions and lymphadenopathy (lymph node enlargement) may occur.
   B. Diagnosis.—RPR or VDRL and darkfield examination of moist lesions.
   C. Treatment.—The same as for primary venereal syphilis.
   D. Alternative treatment.—The same as for primary venereal syphilis.

3. **Early latent venereal syphilis (less than 1 year)**
   A. Symptomology.—None. Approximately 25 percent of patients untreated experience a temporary relapse of primary and secondary syphilitic symptomology during the first 2 years of latent syphilis. The chancre may reappear at its original site and the rash of secondary syphilis may reappear; these symptoms again disappear within a few weeks as systemic disease continues. After 1 year of latent syphilis, most patients are noninfectious except for pregnant women.[1,10,33,46]
   B. Diagnosis.—Positive RPR or VDRL plus positive FTA-ABS or MHA. A history of negative serology or suggestive symptoms within the previous 12 months.
   C. Treatment.—The same as for primary and secondary syphilis.
   D. Alternative treatment.—The same as for primary and secondary syphilis.

4. **Late latent venereal syphilis (greater than 1 year)**
   A. Symptomology.—None.
   B. Diagnosis.—A positive RPR or VDRL plus a positive FTA-ABS or MHA.
   C. Treatment.—Penicillin G Benzathine 2.4 mu/IM weekly for 3 weeks or Penicillin G procaine 600,000 u/IM daily for 15 days.
   D. Alternative Treatment.—Tetracycline HCL 500 mg p.o./q.i.d. for 30 days; Erythromycin 500 mg p.o./q.i.d. for 30 days.

Venereal Syphilis

5. **Cardiovascular tertiary syphilis**
   A. Symptomology. — Evidence of aortitis.
   B. Diagnosis. — A positive RPR or VDRL plus a positive FTA-ABS or MHA. Refer to patient's M.D.
   C. Treatment. — The same as for late latent syphilis.
   D: Alternative Treatment. — The same as for late latent syphilis.

6. **Tertiary venereal neurosyphilis**
   A. Symptomology. — Varied. There may be meningeal, vascular, or parenchymal (tabes or GPI) syndromes; however, the patient may be asymptomatic.
   B. Diagnosis. — Refer the patient for hospitalization; compatible syndrome plus positive serology and abnormal spinal fluid.
   C. Treatment. — Refer the patient for hospitalization; Penicillin G crystalline 24 mu/IV q.i.d. times 10 followed by Penicillin G. Benzathine 2.4 mu/IM weekly for three weeks.
   D. Alternative Treatment. — Penicillin G procaine 600,000 u/IM daily for 15 days, followed by Penicillin G. Benzathine 2.4 mu weekly for 3 weeks. If the patient has a history of an allergy to penicillin, consultation is *strongly advised*.

7. **Early Congenital Venereal Syphilis (under 2 years' duration)**
   A. Symptomology. — Bullous eruptions (most often upon the palms and soles); mucous membrane lesions (snuffles).
   B. Diagnosis. — A positive RPR or VDRL plus a positive FTA-ABS or MHA, darkfield, and CSF examination.
   C. Treatment. — Penicillin G crystalline 50,000 u/kg IM or IV daily in 2 divided dosages for a minimum of 10 days or Penicillin G procaine 50,000 units per kg IM daily for a minimum of 10 days.
   D. Alternative Treatment. — If the patient has a penicillin allergy, consultation is *strongly advised*.

8. **Late Congenital Venereal Syphilis (over 2 years' duration)**
   A. Symptomology. — Interstitial keratitis, "notched" incisors, mulberry molars, bone involvement, deafness.
   B. Diagnosis. — A positive RPR or VDRL plus a positive FTA-ABS or MHA.
   C. Treatment. — After the neonatal period, the same dosage should be utilized as for neonatal congenital syphilis. For larger children, the total dosage needed does not have to exceed the dosage utilized in adult syphilis of more than 1 year's duration.

Note — Follow all patients treated with qualitative and quantitative RPR or VDRL tests. Sexual contacts should be examined and treated. Prompt, efficient epidemiology prevents the spread of infectious syphilis. All infectious syphilis should be immediately reported to the department of health.

The FTA-ABS is more sensitive and more specific that is the VDRL or RPR. Therefore, *a positive RPR or VDRL should be confirmed with the FTA-ABS.* If venereal syphilis is strongly suspected, the FTA-ABS should be performed even if the RPR or VDRL is negative; further, treatment should *not* be delayed while awaiting the FTA-ABS results.

Some medical authorities prefer to treat early syphilis (Primary, secondary, and early latent less than 1 year) with Penicillin G Benzathine 2.4 mu weekly for 2 weeks.

Infants born to women treated for syphilis during pregnancy with erythromycin should be retreated at birth with penicillin.

Note especially the following:

Every patient should have an RPR and complete cultures for gonorrhea; other forms of STD must be given careful consideration with *all* patients.

It is important to remember that females may have double or triple infections so that, for example, the concomitant presence of trichomoniasis and candidiasis may require dual chemotherapy.

If the darkfield examination is positive, treat the patient for syphilis; if negative, treat the patient for syphilis if: (1) The RPR is positive and syphilis is clinically suspected; (2) The RPR is positive and the follow-up is uncertain; and (3) The follow-up is uncertain and syphilis is suspected regardless of the RPR results.

If the darkfield examination is negative and the follow-up is highly unlikely, the patient may be reevaluated without therapy. The RPR should be repeated and an FTA-ABS performed with the patient returning for 2 days for darkfield examination and patient reevaluation within 1 week. Then, if the RPR, FTA-ABS, and the darkfield are all negative, have the patient return within 30 days for an RPR and FTA-ABS. If negative, repeat both of these tests within 60 days.

Jarisch-Herxheimer Reaction

Formerly known as "therapeutic shock," this reaction is believed to be due to the rapid destruction of *T. pallidum* by potent treponemicidal chemotherapeutic agents.[1,46] It is noted following the administration of any treponemicidal agent and is evidence of the medication functioning rather than of an allergic reaction.[46] The reaction generally initiates 6 to 12 hours following chemotherapy and rarely persists beyond 24 hours.[1,33] Reactions may be local or systemic, with many if not most patients being unaware of the reaction.[1,46]

The local reaction consists of an intensification of the lesions. In primary syphilis, the chancre may become edematous, with an increase in size of the satellite bubo (lymph node). A faint secondary rash may become prominent.[33,46] Systemically, the temperature may rise to 102 to 104°F, with such reactions most marked in stages when treponemes are abundant.[46] The reaction is common in early syphilis but is rarely a cause for alarm. Patients should be informed that they may experience this reaction; antipyretics and analgesics help to reduce discomfort.[46]

Generally, the reaction is benign, indicating a favorable response to chemotherapy; however, in late syphilis, the reaction may be more severe.[1,33,46] Regardless of severity, treatment should *not* be discontinued.[46] This reaction must *not* be confused with an allergic reaction. Malaise, headache, and a "general flu-like" feeling is common.[10] Agitation, convulsions, and transient psychosis have been reported in patients with general paresis following the initiation of treatment; however, these reactions are generally brief and rarely necessitate interruption of chemotherapy even in this instance.[1]

Posttreatment Observation for Venereal Syphilis

Approximately 5 percent of the American populus is allergic to penicillin. Generalized urticaria characterized by hives without a shock state may arise from penicillin or other antibiotic administration to which the patient is allergic. Anaphylactoid shock (first exposure to the antigen or drug) and anaphylactic shock (subsequent exposure to the antigen or drug) exists when the following signs and symptoms exist:[1,10,33]

- Tachycardia — Pulse weak and *over 100/min.*
- Systolic blood pressure *under 100 mm Hg.*
- Sudden collapse
- Heachache and/or "ringing in the ears"
- Erythema (redness) and pruritus (itching) of the skin; particularly of the face and chest
- Edema (swelling) of the face, hands, feet, ear lobes, tongue, etc.
- Angioneurotic and/or pulmonary edema
- Abdominal pain
- Nausea/vomiting
- Weakness
- Wheezing and/or sneezing
- History of previous allergic response
- Respiratory efforts shallow/irregular

The treatment for such reactions is epinephrine 1:1,000 .3 mg SQ and benedryl 25-50 mg IV push along with oxygen and other care procedures to combat shock as necessary (MAST trousers, IV's of lactated ringer's solution or normal saline solution, and vasopressors).[1,33]

All patients should be closely observed for at least 20 minutes following penicillkin injection, and careful preparations made beforehand in anticipation of emergencies.[1,10,33,46]

Following the completion of treatment, patients should return each month during the first year for quantitative serologic tests and examination for relapsing lesions.[33] Should the patient develop a recurrence of primary/secondary symptoms, if there is evidence of tertiary syphilis, or following the birth of a syphilitic infant, retreatment is necessary.[33]

If the STS in patients with early syphilis shows no appreciable decrease within 6 months or if the titer is elevated (arbitrarily a dilution of 1:4 or higher) one year after chemotherapy, further treatment is indicated.[1,33] A positive reaction in any dilution 18 months or more after treatment of primary or secondary syphilis should be considered a treatment failure and another course of chemotherapy administered.[1,33]

Relapse and Reinfection

Evidence of relapse in early syphilis may arise as early as 4 weeks or as late as 2 years post-treatment.[1,33] The prognosis of relapsing venereal syphilis is more serious than an initial infection, and retreatment with twice the original dosage of penicillin is indicated, given over a longer period of time.[1,33] Many patients with recurrent syphilis actually have a new infection rather than a relapse of their original infection.[33] Although various criteria have been established to distinguish a relapse from reinfection, differentiation is often impossible.[33]

20. Viral Hepatitis Infections

Viral hepatitis is an acute systemic infectious disease predominantly affecting the liver as an acute inflammation with temporary necrosis (destruction) of liver cells. The disease occurs in two epidemiologically distinct but clinically similar forms: infectious hepatitis (hepatitis A) and serum hepatitis (hepatitis B).[1,6,8,10,33,35] While viral hepatitis is not strictly a sexually transmitted disease, both forms of hepatitis may be acquired through the medium of sexual contact.[12,35] Both forms are characterized pathologically by hepatic cell necrosis and clinically by a grippe-like syndrome, jaundice, and subsequent recovery, with many asymptomatic cases reported through abnormal liver function tests.[1,33]

Occurrence

Hepatitis B has emerged as a significant sexually transmitted disease among gay and bisexual males; approximately 60 percent of all cases of hepatitis B infection occur among this population.[10,34,35] Preliminary data from selected homosexual groups indicate that approximately 10 percent of uninfected patients will become infected with hepatitis B each year. Studies of selected populations indicate that approximately 50 percent of gay males may have the antibody to hepatitis B virus, indicating past infection with hepatitis.[34]

The American Public Health Association notes that infectious hepatitis (A) occurs worldwide sporadically and in epidemics, with outbreaks most common in institutions, rural regions, and military forces during wartime. The disease is most common among children and young adults and less prevalent with advancing years; the seasonal incidence is highest in autumn and early winter in temperate zones. Serum hepatitis (B) has a worldwide distribution, with a prevalence among recipients of pooled blood products varying from 0.1 percent to 12 percent, with known icterogenic plasma as high as 60 percent.[6]

Infectious Etiological Agents

The infectious etiological agents for hepatitis A and B are DNA viruses with antigenic components known as hepatitis B virus (HBV) and hepatitis A virus (HAV).[12,35] Although the precise size of the infectious hepatitis virus (HAV) is idiopathic, the serum hepatitis virus (HBV) has been postulated upon the basis of filtration studies to be less than 26 mu in diameter. Both agents resist freezing for months and are not destroyed by heating at 56°C for one-half hour. The serum hepatitis virus is inactivated by heating at 60°C for 10 hours, and the infectious hepatitis virus is probably also susceptible to such treatment. Both viruses are resistant to ether; the infectious hepatitis virus remains infective following exposure to chlorine (1 part per million).[33] Infectious agents which may cause hepatitis include viruses, spirochetes, protozoa, and bacteria.[1] Toxic agents which may cause hepatitis include carbon tetrachloride and other industrial solvents, phosphorus, anesthetic agents, antibiotics, and psychopharmacologic agents.[1,33]

Reservoir and Source of Infection

The reservoir is mankind; perhaps rarely chimpanzees. Sources of infection are feces, and bodily fluids from infected persons. Presence of the infectious agent in the nasopharynx is not proved but commonly assumed upon epidemiologic grounds.[6]

Mode of Transmission

To date, all of the modes of transmission for viral hepatitis have not been identified. Infectious hepatitis A is most commonly associated with fecal-oral contamination from person-to-person contact, from sewage-contaminated foods, whole blood transfusions, and contaminated syringes, with respiratory spread possible.[6,35] Serum hepatitis, or hepatitis B, can be transmitted sexually as this virus is present (as is the virus of hepatitis A) in seminal fluid, urine, feces, saliva, and vaginal secretions.[29,35] Traditionally, this disease was believed to be most commonly transmitted parenterally (intravenously, intramuscularly, or subcutaneously) by inoculation of human blood, plasma, serum, or thrombin from an infected person or by utilization of contaminated syringes or other instruments.[6] Immune (gamma) globulin and heat-treated albumin, although blood derivatives, do not transmit the disease.[6]

Incubation Period

The incubation period for viral hepatitis varies from 12 days to 6 months.[1,6,11,33] The incubation period for hepatitis A varies between 15 to 60 days, irrespective of the route of inoculation, and in most epidemics averages approximately 30 days.[33] The incubation period for hepatitis B is longer, with a range of 60 to 180 days, but generally, 80 to 100 days.[6,33]

Period of Communicability

Studies show that the viral hepatitis patient may be infectious long before the onset of symptomology and long after clinical manifestations disappear. Patients who are asymptomatic may be just as infectious as symptomatic patients.[11] Clinical experience with hepatitis A suggests that the period of greatest communicability is from several days before to generally not more than 7 days after the onset of manifest disease. For hepatitis B, infectiousness exists from at least 89 days before symptomology appears to be at least 8 days following the onset of jaundice.[6]

Susceptibility and Resistance

Hepatitis virus B infections are more common in gay and bisexual men than in heterosexual males; a recent study showed that 50 percent of homosexual males tested had previously been exposed to the virus, as compared to less than 11 percent of the heterosexual men.[11] The degree of immunity following an attack of disease is idiopathic. Second attacks may occur, but second attacks of jaundice are rare.[6]

Gamma globulin given soon after exposure to hepatitis may reduce the risks of infection if administered promptly.[11] Such injections of gamma globulin are of no value once manifest disease has occurred.[1,11,33]

An effective vaccine has been developed for hepatitis virus B infections and is presently being utilized and retested at this time.[11]

Signs and Symptoms

1. Asymptomatic cases.—For every clinical case of hepatitis, there appear to be several asymptomatic or subclinical cases of hepatitis within the community. Such asymptomatic carriers of infection may readily transmit this disease to others.[1,11]

2. Flu-like symptoms.—The disease typically begins with flu-like symptoms of lassitude, weakness, drowsiness, anorexia, nausea, vomiting, abdominal pain, fever, and headache.[1]

3. Jaundice does not always occur, but when it does, it typically follows the flu-like symptoms and lasts for approximately 2 weeks.[1,33]

4. Dark urine, gray stools, and mild pruritus are commonly reported in conjunction with jaundice.[1]

5. Tender hypertrophied liver and/or spleen is a common finding in many cases.

6. Lymphadenopathy and spider angiomas may occur with hepatitis; most commonly, the lymphadenopathy is posterior-cervical in nature.[1]

Diagnosis

The diagnosis of viral hepatitis is by medical history, clinical manifestations noted upon physical examination, and laboratory tests of liver damage.[11] The single most valuable test is the serum transaminase (SGOT, SGPT), which can be expected to rise several days prior to the onset of jaundice. Positive tests for hepatitis surface antigen (HBsAG) indicate an acute HBV infection, or without acute disease exposure, a chronic carrier state. Positive tests for HBe antigen indicate current infectiousness, while anti-HBsAG indicates past infection with present immunity and anti-HB core antigen indicates past or current infection.[12]

Treatment

There is no specific therapy; supportive therapy should be provided by a physician. Rest, excellent diet, and avoidance of liver toxins such as alcohol and most drugs constitute the treatment of this disease.[1,11] Complete recovery may require many months, with chemotherapy in the form of prednisone or other drugs sometimes prescribed.

21. Yaws

Yaws is an acute and chronic infectious tropical disease caused by *Treponema pertenue*. The disease is characterized by a primary cutaneous lesion followed by a granulomatous skin eruption, and in some instances, by late destructive lesions of the skin and bones.[1,33] Synonyms for this disease include *frambesia tropica, pian, bouba, parangi, pain,* and many others.[6,33]

Occurrence

Yaws is primarily a disease of rural tropics and subtropics, with the lowest socioeconomic groups having the highest rates.[6] It is primarily a childhood disease, but it may occur at any age, with males outnumbering females.[6] Yaws is most prevalent in the West Indies, South Pacific islands, equatorial Africa, and Indonesia, with endemic foci in Caribbean areas, parts of Brazil, Columbia, Venezuela, Peru, Ecuador, Panama, and British Guiana. Incidence is decreasing in many regions.[6,33]

Infectious Etiological Agent

Yaws is caused by *Treponema pertenue*, morphologically indistinguishable from *Treponema pallidum*, which causes veneral syphilis.[8,33] It further resembles the spirochete of syphilis in that it produces a positive reaction with serological tests for syphilis (STS) with the same frequency as for syphilis, becoming positive during the initial stage, remaining positive during the early stage, and becoming nonreactive again after many years of latency, even without specific treatment.[1,6,10,33]

Reservoir and Source of Infection

The reservoir is mankind; the source of infection is exudates of early skin lesions of infected persons.[6,33]

Mode of Transmission

Some authorities consider yaws to be a sexually transmitted disease, while others do not. The disease is communicated primarily via direct contact; indirect transmission by contaminated articles and flies is uncertain and probably of minor significance.[6] Transmission of this disease rarely occurs by sexual contact.[33]

Incubation Period

The incubation period for yaws is from 2 weeks to 3 months.[1,6,8,33] An initial lesion most typically appears within 3 to 6 weeks, generally followed by mild constitutional symptoms within several weeks to months of infectious onset, often prior to the healing of the primary lesion.[6]

Period of Communicability

The period of communicability for yaws is variable. It may extend intermittently over several years while relapsing moist lesions are present.[6] The infectious agent is not generally found in late ulcerative lesions.[6]

Susceptibility and Resistance

There is no evidence of a natural or racial resistance for this disease. Infection results in immunity to homologous and heterologous strains, of slower evolution for heterologous strains and probably not complete until 1 year. The part of superinfection in nature is not well defined and may be unimportant.[6] Cross immunity between syphilis and yaws has been observed in both mankind and experimental animals. The disease is more common among natives with poor personal hygiene habits.[33]

Signs and Symptoms

1. **Primary lesion** (the mother yaw) appears at the site of inoculation, which is almost invariably extragenital and generally occurs upon the legs. The lesion is a granuloma, which later ulcerates and heals with scar formation.[33]

2. **Generalized eruption** occurs approximately 6 to 12 weeks following lesion appearance, consisting of large papules or granulomas upon the face, neck, extremities, and buttocks.[1,33] These lesions commonly occur about the mucocutaneous junctions, such as the mouth, nose, and rectum,

and resemble the condylomas of secondary syphilis.[36] They heal slowly. Relapses may occur months or years following the onset of the initial yaw.[33] The lesions of yaws often appear upon the soles of the feet and produce painful ulcerations known as crab yaws.[33]

3. Late manifestations of disease appear after several years, consisting of late destructive lesions in the skin and bones. Periostitis and osteitis are found in the bones of the hands, arms, and legs, producing characteristic dactylitis and "saber shins." Destructive lesions appear about the nose and result in severe ulcerative areas (gangosa).[33] Proliferative exostoses develop in the nasal portion of the maxillary bones; this is known as goundou.[33] Juxtaarticular nodules are also seen in the late stage of this disease. Involvement of the aorta and the central nervous system have been reported as complications in rare instances.[33]

Diagnosis

A presumptive diagnosis can often be made upon the appearance of the generalized skin eruption alone, but *T. pertenue* is easily demonstrated in the lesions.[33] The darkfield and STS are generally positive.[33] The lesions of yaws may be confused with those of leishmaniasis, leprosy, tuberculosis, and late gummatous syphilis.[33]

Treatment

Penicillin is the drug of choice, producing prompt disappearance of treponemes on darkfield examination and rapid healing of lesions.[1,33] The recommended dosage is 1.2 million units of procaine penicillin in adults with early active lesions and less for children and latent cases.[33] Tetracycline may be utilized for this disease but is generally less preferred than penicillin.[33]

22. Toward the Prevention and Control of the Sexually Transmitted Diseases

There are many reasons for the persistence of sexually transmitted diseases (STDs) as a common and significant health threat to those residing within the United States and throughout the world. Some of these reasons are as follows:[10,11,14,35,83]

- Patients often do not know the symptoms of STDs, where to get accurate information concerning these diseases, and where to get treatment when infected.
- Patients often are too embarrassed or afraid to seek help due to parental attitudes toward such diseases. Young people may not know that they can be treated without parental consent in virtually every state within the United States.
- Upon discovering their infection, people may not appreciate the need to inform sexual contacts, or may be too embarrassed to do so. Sexual contacts that are unknown to the patient cannot be informed that they may have an STD.
- There are a large number of asymptomatic carriers for many forms of STD.
- It appears that people are becoming more sexually active at younger ages with the change in social mores and improved methods of contraception. These young people may be uneducated regarding STDs.
- Birth control pills themselves increase a woman's chances of contracting gonorrhea from approximately 50 percent to 100 percent; in addition, utilization of the pill eliminates condom use, which significantly increases the degree of communicability for many forms of sexually transmitted disease.
- Sexually transmitted diseases often remain communicable for extended periods of time and may be communicable prior to the onset of clinical manifestations.
- There is no simple blood test for many forms of STD such as

gonorrhea; patients may be reluctant to specify the need for other diagnostic tests such as pharyngeal, rectal, cervical, and urethral cultures.
- There is no vaccine for most forms of sexually transmitted disease. Vaccination may represent the only ultimate cure for the persistent epidemic of gonorrhea and other STDs within the United States and throughout the world.
- Many forms of STD are highly communicable, as in the case of condyloma acuminata, herpes progenitalis, viral hepatitis, secondary syphilis, and others.
- There is no acquired immunity for sexually transmitted diseases in general.
- There are technological problems of bacterial resistance, ineffective chemotherapy for STDs caused by viruses, and false-negative test results.
- There is often a general lack of concern among the public for those afflicted with such diseases.
- Some professionals do not possess a current and thorough knowledge concerning the nature, diagnosis, and appropriate treatment for such diseases; as such, some patients will receive incomplete and inappropriate treatment for STD.
- Frequently, little if any accurate information is presented on STDs within public and private schools, particularly in regard to diseases other than gonorrhea and syphilis.

The following suggestions have been made by a variety of medical authorities to reduce or potentially reduce the spread of sexually transmitted diseases.[1,10,11,34]

- Avoid promiscuous sexual behavoir. While some forms of sexually transmitted disease can be contracted nonsexually, generally these diseases are communicated by sexual contact and are most prevalent among those who are promiscuous, particularly with anonymous sexual partners. Avoid sex with the promiscuous as well.
- Utilize a condom. Condom use can be of significant benefit in reducing the degree of communicability for many forms of STD, along with reducing the probability of an unwanted pregnancy.
- Utilize birth control foams or Certa Foam. Birth control foams and Certa Foam (developed by the University of Pittsburgh Medical Center) may reduce the probability of contracting some forms of STD by 50 percent or more.
- Have periodic medical examinations and laboratory tests. Individuals who are highly sexually active should be examined approximately every 6 months and should have a serology for syphilis and complete cultures.
- Urinate and shower following sexual activity. These two simple

measures may be of some benefit in reducing the contraction probabilities for a number of sexually transmitted diseases.

- Seek immediate treatment for STD symptomology. Individuals must know the clinical manifestations for STD and monitor themselves for such; upon recognition of STD symptomology, immediate treatment and avoidance of sexual activity until cure is apparent is the appropriate course of action.
- Know and inform sexual contacts if infected. In consideration of one's sexual partner(s), one should avoid sex if infected and immediately inform sexual contacts so that they may be immediately treated as well.
- Wash clothing and bedding regularly. Be sure to properly decontaminate underwear, bedding, etc., which may be infested with itch mites or pubic lice.
- Avoid self-treatment for sexually transmitted diseases. With the exception of pediculosis pubis infestation, one should not attempt self-treatment for STDs.
- Obtain STD vaccines when available. As vaccines become available for more forms of STD, these should be obtained, particularly by those who constitute a population at risk.
- Support health education within our schools. Be sure that local school systems include current, comprehensive, and nonjudgmental information concerning STDs.
- Avoid the utilization of drugs related to STDs such as intravenous utilization of drugs, isobutyl nitrite, amyl nitrite, etc.
- Attempt to maintain general good health. Obtain sufficient rest and sleep; avoid and reduce stress, practice excellent personal hygiene, and engage in good nutrition practices. Take all medications as prescribed unless an allergic reaction becomes apparent, in which case the medication should be immediately discontinued and the prescribing physician consulted at once.
- Medical authorities also urge reporting of STD cases by physicians and vigorous contact-finding when possible.

In most states, minors may be treated for sexually transmitted diseases without parental consent; however, if child abuse is suspected, health personnel have an obligation to report it to CHILDLINE at 1-800-932-0313. The law provides immunity for good-faith reporting in all states. The nearest clinic may be located by calling Operation Venus at 1-800-462-4966, the National VD Hotline at 1-800-227-8922, or the State Health Hotline at 1-800-692-7254, all of which are toll-free calls.[11]

Some STD patients for many reasons may be unable to inform their sexual partners of their diagnosis of STD; fortunately, there are alternatives. Health departments typically employ "public health representatives" who can locate these sexual partners and arrange for definitive diagnosis and treatment. Sexual partners are not informed of the patient's

Prevention and Control

name or any other identifying information about the patient who has identified them as a sexual contact.[11]

Ideally, if vaccines could be developed for all forms of sexually transmitted disease and administered in infancy and early childhood along with other "baby shots," and if lifelong immunity to all forms of STD were provided by such, then all forms of sexually transmissible disease might be eradicated. However, the reality is that to date, only one vaccine, effective against hepatitis virus B infection, has been developed.[11]

For those who suffer from immunodeficiency, Roger W. Enlow, M.D., offers the following advice:[73]

- Avoid unnecessary exposure, especially intimate contact with people who have colds or flu or who do not feel well. The viruses which cause colds or flu are transmitted by contact with saliva or mucous secretions from the infected person until he or she is well.

- Minor injuries such as cuts and abrasions should be promptly cleaned with soap and water and then covered with a sterile dressing and bandage to prevent the entry of germs, many kinds of which are common in our everyday environment. Injuries that do not heal well should be reported to your physician promptly; the physician can prescribe antibiotic chemotherapy and other needed treatment to help cure infection and promote healing.

- Limit the number of sexual partners whose health status is questionable or unknown. This means fewer sexual partners and avoidance of individuals who have a large variety of sexual partners themselves. Sexual encounters should be avoided in such places as baths, "back rooms," movie theaters, etc., as sexual partners in such places tend to comprise a population at risk for sexually transmitted diseases.

- Some sexual activities may be more risky than others, particularly with sexual partners whose identity is unknown. These include ingestion of seminal fluid or urine, oral-anal sexual contact, or any other activity in which there is fecal-oral contact.

- Be sure that your physician knows that you have an immune deficiency disease prior to accepting any form of vaccination. Many vaccines are composed of attenuated (altered but living) organisms, which will not generally harm individuals with normal immune capabilities but might represent a life-threatening problem for the immune deficient.

- Avoid travel to regions of the world where diseases such as amebiasis, giardia, malaria, or typhoid fever are common. These diseases may cause special problems for AIDS patients and others with various forms of immune deficiency.

- Be sure that fruits and vegetables are well washed or peeled. Some molds and fungus infections may be present on the outside and may provide infectious disease.

- Be sure that meats are well-cooked, especially beef, which occasionally contains pathogenic microorganisms.

- Avoid exposure to dusty environments, particularly where animals (including birds) have lived. In such environments, many potentially pathogenic microorganisms can be inhaled, ingested, or contracted through skin lesions. In addition, some domestic new pets, including birds, cats, and dogs, may not be well and should be examined by a veterinarian prior to accepting them as a part of one's family. Even then, careful disposal of animal feces and urine is important.
- Avoid the excessive utilization of antibiotics. Take them only when a physician directs you to do so. Pathogenic microorganisms may develop a resistance to antibiotics taken repeatedly, which makes the overutilization of such drugs dangerous. Physicians can perform cultures to definitively diagnose many forms of infection and then select the best form of chemotherapy for the disease. Antibiotics in general do nothing for viral infections and many only make things worse (except for some newer antiviral antibiotics).
- Eat a balanced, nutritious diet with a full measure of vitamins, minerals, proteins, carbohydrates, fats, water, and roughage. While some individuals believe that extreme dietary regimens have preventive or therapeutic value, these claims are generally unproven medically.
- Under no circumstance should drugs be taken intravenously unless supervised by a physician aware of your immune deficiency, as I.V. drug abuse constitutes a major risk factor for AIDS, hepatitis, and a variety of other life-threatening conditions such as emboli, septicemia, and street market toxicity, even in individuals with uncompromised immune system functioning. Certain steroids taken intramuscularly may be harmful to the immune system as well.
- Recreational drug utilization, while examined in many AIDS studies, remains of idiopathic harm; some drugs have been utilized for thousands of years by many different cultures, while others are comparatively recent and less familiar to us. A reduction in recreational drug utilization is definitely warranted until more is known about AIDS and immune deficiency syndromes in general.
- Avoid utilizing other people's toothbrush and razor in particular; have your own to protect yourself and others. Some medical authorities recommend keeping disposable razors in a glass of alcohol, with careful washing upon utilization to prevent certain forms of dermatitis.
- If your physician has informed you that your platelet count is low, be cautious should you cut yourself, applying direct pressure to control hemorrhaging. Be careful in participating in activities where injuries are likely. Avoid aspirin-containing products; read labels to be sure, since aspirin further decreases the effectiveness of platelet clotting.
- Ask your dentist whether you should have antibiotics before or after dental treatment.
- Reduce stress within your life and *take better care of yourself*! Don't push to the last ounce of energy—pace yourself. When tired, pay attention to your body by resting and relaxing. Get adequate sleep and learn

to say "no" when you need to rest. When you wake up tired, get more rest and sleep.

Educational Activities

The Centers for Disease Control in Atlanta, Georgia, have noted that the primary purpose of STD education is to complement and support efforts to control the sexually transmitted diseases. As such, notes the CDC, educational activities represent an intregral aspect of public health control programs and need to be thoroughly integrated into all strata of society if control of these diseases is to be achieved.[34]

The concept of integrated activities is central to a comprehensive policy statement developed by a special work group of CDC's Veneral Disease Control Division in 1977. Copies of *VD Guidelines: Education* have been distributed to state and local health departments throughout the United States and are available from state health departments and the CDC.

The guidelines delineate 4 broad target populations at whom educational efforts are being directed:[34]

1. Patients infected with one or more sexually transmitted diseases.

2. Providers delivering any level of care to STD patients.

3. Special groups having indentifiable characteristics, including a significant risk of acquiring infection.

4. General public, whose support is essential to control efforts.

In addition to suggesting techniques and measures appropriate to each target population, the guidelines emphasize the importance of setting specific, measurable objectives and of evaluating educational efforts upon the basis of their value in disease intervention.[34]

Today more than ever, ignorance, arrogance, and hypocrisy concerning the sexually transmitted diseases are to be repudiated.[73] The magnitude of the problem of sexually transmitted diseases within the United States and throughout the world is astounding. The opportunity for promotion of health and prevention of human suffering, societal costs, and death from sexually transmitted diseases is our challenge.[14]

References

1. Robert Berkow, M.D., editor. *The Merck Manual of Diagnosis and Therapy*. Rahway, N.J.: Merck Sharp and Dohme Research Laboratories, 1981.
2. Clarence W. Tabor. *Taber's Cyclopedic Medical Dictionary*. 11th ed. Philadelphia: F.A. Davis, 1970.
3. Wesley Alles, Ph.D., and Laurna Rubinson, Ph.D. *Health Education—Foundations for the Future*. St. Louis: Times-Mirror/Mosby College, 1984.
4. Herpes Resource Center. *Herpes Alert*. Palo Alto, Calif.: Herpes Resource Center, 1983.
5. James L. McCary, Ph.D. *Human Sexuality—A Brief Edition*. New York: Van Nostrand, 1973.
6. M. D. Beneson, editor, and others. *The Control of Communicable Diseases in Man*. 13th ed. New York: American Public Health Association, 1981.
7. Benjamin Kogan, M.D., D.P.H. *Health in a Changing Environment*. 2nd ed. New York: Harcourt Brace Jovanovich, 1974.
8. Marion E. Wilson, Ph.D. *Microbiology in Patient Care*. 2nd ed. New York: Macmillan, 1976.
9. Communicable Disease Centers. *Sexually Transmitted Disease Statistical Letter*. Atlanta: Communicable Disease Centers and U.S. Department of Health and Human Services, 1982.
10. Donna Cherniak and Allan Feingold. *The Venereal Disease Handbook*. Canada: 1975.
11. Pennsylvania Department of Health, Division of Acute Infectious Diseases. *Resource Guide on Sexually Transmitted Diseases*. Harrisburg, Pa.: Pennsylvania Department of Health, 1982.
12. Communicable Disease Centers, Technical Information Services, Center for Prevention Services. *Sexually Transmitted Disease Summary—1982*. Atlanta: Communicable Disease Centers, 1982.
13. Barbara J. Combs, and others. *An Invitation to Health*, Menlo Park, Calif.: Benjamin-Cummings, 1983.
14. Paul J. Wiesner, M.D. *Magnitude of the Problem of Sexually Transmitted Diseases in the United States*. Atlanta: U.S. Department of Health and Human Services, Public Health Service, Centers for Disease Control, 1980.
15. Centers for Disease Control, U.S. Public Health Service. "Statistics on Sexually Transmitted Diseases—AIDS—1984." Time (April 30, 1984):66–67.
16. E. R. Mahoney, Ph.D. *Human Sexuality*. New York: McGraw-Hill, 1983.
17. James L. McCary, Ph.D. and Stephen P. McCary, Ph.D. *McCary's Human Sexuality*. 4th ed. Belmont, Calif.: Wadsworth, 1982.
18. M. F. Rein, M.D. "Therapeutic Decisions in the Treatment of Sexually Transmitted Diseases—An Overview." *Sexually Transmitted Diseases—Journal of the American Venereal Disease Association* 8 (1981).

References

19. Laurene Mascola, M.D., M.P.H., and others. "Gonorrhea in American Teenagers, 1960 to 1981." U.S. Public Health Service, Centers for Disease Control, and *Pediatric Infectious Disease* 2, no. 4 (1983).

20. Akbar A. Zaidi, M.D., and others. "Gonorrhea in the United States: 1967-1979." *Sexually Transmitted Diseases — Journal of the American Venereal Disease Association* 10, no. 2 (April-June, 1983).

21. Pennsylvania Department of Health, Division of Acute Infectious Diseases. *Statistics on Sexually Transmitted Diseases*. Harrisburg, Pa.: 1984.

22. Communicable Disease Centers, U.S. Public Health Service. *Sexually Transmitted Disease (STD) Statistical Newsletter*. Washington, D.C.: U.S. Department of Health and Human Services, 1984.

23. Joseph Chiappa, director for Sexually Transmitted Disease Education, Philadelphia Department of Public Health, Philadelphia, Pa.

24. William Boyd, M.D. *An Introduction to the Study of Disease*. 6th ed. Philadelphia: Lea and Febiger, 1971.

25. University of Pittsburgh Medical Center. *Research on Sexually Transmitted Diseases*. Pittsburgh, Pa.

26. Philadelphia Department of Health, Division of Sexually Transmitted Diseases. *Statistics on Sexually Transmitted Diseases*. Philadelphia: 1984.

27. Centers for Disease Control, U.S. Public Health Service. *Survey of Research on Sexually Transmitted Diseases*. Washington, D.C.: U.S. Department of Health and Human Services, 1984.

28. T. Rosen, M.D. "Unusual Presentations of Gonorrhea." *Journal of The American Academy of Dermatology* 6, no. 3 (March, 1982).

29. National Institutes of Health, The U.S. Public Health Service. *Sexually Transmitted Diseases*. Maryland: National Institute of Allergy and Infectious Diseases, 1976.

30. American Social Health Association. *Venereal Disease: Getting the Right Answers*. Palo Alto, Calif.: 1977.

31. Andrew H. Rudolph, M.D. "Stopping the Spread of Gonorrhea." *Hospital Medicine* (January, 1972).

32. Edward B. Johns, Ed.D. *Health for Effective Living*. 6th ed. New York: McGraw-Hill, 1975.

33. Kurt Isselbacker, and others. *Harrison's Principles of Internal Medicine*. 9th ed. New York: McGraw-Hill, 1980.

34. Centers for Disease Control, U.S. Public Health Service. *STD Fact Sheet*. 34th ed. Atlanta: Centers for Disease Control, 1981.

35. Gay Men's Health Project. *Health and Venereal Disease Guide for Gay Men*. New York: Gay Men's Health Project, 1982.

36. Charles Rinear, Ed.D. *The Sexually Transmitted Diseases*. Unpublished manuscript (Summer, 1974).

37. Nathan Fain. "Is Our Lifestyle Hazardous to Our Health?" *The Advocate* (March 18, 1982).

38. Mark Freedman, Ph.D. *Loving Man*. New York: Hark, 1976.

39. Pennsylvania Department of Public Health, Division of Acute Infectious Diseases. *Sexually Transmitted Diseases: Diagnostic Approach, Specific Diagnosis, and Recommended Therapy*. Harrisburg, Pa.: Pennsylvania Department of Public Health, September 1982.

40. American Cancer Society.*Cancer Facts and Figures — 1984*. New York: American Cancer Society, 1984.

41. Charles Rinear, Ed.D. "An Epidemiological and Attitudinal Analysis of Rape and Other Sexual Assault Among Urban Female Hospital Personnel." Ed. D. Thesis, Pennsylvania State University, 1977.

References

42. Centers for Disease Control and MEDCOM Pharmaceutical Corporation. *Criteria and Techniques for the Diagnosis and Treatment of Gonorrhea and Syphilis.* Atlanta: 1974.

43. Leslie Nicholas, M.D., professor of Medicine at Hahnamann University Medical Center, Philadelphia, Pa.

44. Herant Katchadourian, M.D., and Donald T. Lunde, M.D. *Fundamentals of Human Sexuality.* 2nd ed. New York: Holt, Rinehart and Winston, 1975.

45. U.S. Department of Health and Human Services, U.S. Public Health Service. *Strictly for Teenagers — Some Facts About Venereal Disease.* Washington, D.C.: U.S. Government Printing Office, Public Health Service Publication Number 913.

46. CIBA Pharmaceutical Company. *Clinical Symposia on Venereal Syphilis* 23, no. 3. Summit, N.J.: CIBA Pharmaceutical Company, Division of CIBA-GEIGY Corporation, 1971.

47. Paul Woolley, M.D., M.P.H., professor of Public Health, Pennsylvania State University.

48. Reed and Carnrick Pharmaceutical Corporation. *What to Do When You're Bugged by Phthirus Pubis.* Kenilworth, N.J.: Reed and Carnrick Pharmaceutical Corporation, 1983.

49. C.B. Schofield. "Some Factors Affecting the Incubation Period and Duration of Symptoms of Urethritis in Men." *The British Journal of Venereal Disease* 58, no. 3 (April-June, 1982).

50. James Lynch, M.D., professor of Psychiatry, University of Maryland Medical Center, Baltimore, Md.

51. Jerome Goldstein, M.D., P.C., professor of Medicine, Hahnamann University Medical College, Philadelphia, Pa.

52. Michael F. Rein, M.D., and Thomas A. Chapel, M.D. "Trichomoniasis, Candidiasis, and the 'Minor' Venereal Diseases." *Clinical Obstetrics and Gynecology* 18, no. 1 (March, 1975).

53. William M. McCormack, M.D. "Sexually Transmissible Conditions Other than Gonorrhea and Syphilis." *The Practice of Medicine*, Vol. III, chapter 20. 1974.

54. American Academy of Dermatology. *Facts About Herpes Simplex.* Evanston, Ill.: American Academy of Dermatology, 1982.

55. American Social Health Association. *Some Questions and Answers About Herpes.* Palo Alto, Calif.: American Social Health Association.

56. M. Guinan, M.D., Ph.D. "The Course of Untreated Recurrent Genital Herpes Simplex Infection." *New England Journal of Medicine* (March 26, 1981): 304.

57. Elena J. Bettoli, R.N., B.S.N., and Mary Guinan, M.D., Ph.D. "Herpes: Facts and Fallacies." *American Journal of Nursing* (June, 1982).

58. Herpes Resource Center. *Herpes Alert.* Palo Alto, Calif.: Herpes Resource Center, 1983.

59. Centers for Disease Control, U.S. Public Health Service. *Herpes Genital Infection.* Atlanta: Centers for Disease Control, 1984.

60. Lawrence Corey, M.D. "The Diagnosis and Treatment of Genital Herpes." *Journal of the American Medical Association* 248, no. 9 (September 3, 1982).

61. Centers for Disease Control, U.S. Public Health Service. *Ineffective Therapies for Genital Herpes Infections.* Atlanta: Centers for Disease Control, 1984.

62. C. McCoy, M.D., and others. "Condyloma Acuminata: An Unusual Presentation of Child Abuse." *Journal of Pediatric Surgery* 17, no. 5 (October, 1982).

63. G. Ejeckam, and others. "Malignant Transformation in an Anal Condyloma Acuminatum." *Canadian Journal of Surgery* 26, no. 2 (March, 1983).

64. American Academy of Dermatology and American Medical Association. *A Dermatologist Talks About Warts.* Evanston, Ill.: American Academy of Dermatology, 1982.

65. S.A. Spector, M. Tyndall, and others. "Effects of Acyclovir Combined with Other Antiviral Agents upon Human Cytomegalovirus Infections." *American Journal of Medicine* 73, no. 1A (July 20, 1982).

66. S. Saigal, M.D., and others. "The Outcome in Children with Congenital Cytomegalovirus Infection." *American Journal of Diseases in Children* 136, no. 10 (October, 1982).

67. W. Knowles, M.D., and others. "A Comparison of Cervical Cytomegalovirus (CMV) Excretion in Gynecological Patients and Postpartum Women." *Archives of Virology* 73, no. 1 (1982).

68. R. Pass, M.D., and others. "Excretion of Cytomegalovirus in Mothers: Observations after Delivery of Congenitally Infected and Normal Infants." *Journal of Infectious Diseases* 146, no. 1 (July, 1982).

69. M.L. Kumar, M.D., and others. "Experimental Primary Cytomegalovirus Infection in Pregnancy: Time and Fetal Outcome." *American Journal of Obstetrics and Gynecology* 145, no. 1 (January 1, 1983).

70. Helen Ortega, M.S., and others. "Enteric Protozoa in Homosexual Men from San Francisco." *Journal of the American Venereal Disease Association* 11, no. 2 (April–June, 1984).

71. Edward Rubenstein, M.D. *Scientific American Medicine.* New York: Scientific American, 1984.

72. D.H. Jackson, M.D. "Carriage and Transmission of Group B Streptococci Among STD Patients." *British Journal of Venereal Disease* 58, no. 5 (October, 1982).

73. Gay Men's Health Crisis. *Acquired Immune Deficiency Syndrome.* New York: Gay Men's Health Crisis, 1983.

74. Anthony S. Fauci, M.D., and others. "Acquired Immunodeficiency Syndrome: Epidemiologic, Clinical, Immunologic, and Therapeutic Considerations." *Annals of Internal Medicine* 100 (January, 1984).

75. Mary E. Guinan, M.D., Ph.D. "Heterosexual and Homosexual Patients with Acquired Immunodeficiency Syndrome." *Annals of Internal Medicine* 100 (February, 1984).

76. Centers for Disease Control. "Acquired Immune Deficiency Syndrome: The Past as Prologue." *Annals of Internal Medicine* 98, no. 3 (March, 1983).

77. Susan West. "One Step Behind a Killer." *Science* (March, 1983).

78. F. Civantos and others. "Kaposi's Sarcoma: Absence of Cytomegalovirus Antigens." *Journal of Investigative Dermatology* 79, no. 2 (August, 1982).

79. E.O. Rasmussen, M.D., and others. "Immunosupression in a Homosexual Man with Kaposi's Sarcoma." *Journal of the American Academy of Dermatology* 6, no. 5 (May, 1982).

80. E. DeStefano, M.D., and others. "Acid-Labile Human Leukocyte Interferon in Homosexual Men with Kaposi's Sarcoma and Lymphadenopathy." *Journal of Infectious Diseases* 146, no. 4 (October, 1982).

81. G.T. Vanley, M.D., and others. "Atypical Pneumocystis Carinii Pneumonia in Homosexual Men with Unusual Immunodeficiency." *American Journal of Research* 138, no. 6 (June, 1982).

82. D. Mildvan, M.D., and others. "Opportunistic Infections and Immune Deficiency in Homosexual Men." *Annals of Internal Medicine* 96, no. 6 (June, 1982).

References

83. University of Pennsylvania Student Health Service. *Acquired Immune Deficiency Syndrome — What All Students Should Know*. Philadelphia: University of Pennsylvania, 1986.

84. Susan West. "AIDS Update — Lots of Leads, Few Answers." *Science '83*, (October, 1983): 16-18.

85. J. Post. "What Do We Know About AIDS?" *Family Life Educator* 2 (Winter, 1983): 10-11.

86. M. Hamrick and others. *Health*. Columbus, Ohio: Merrill, 1986.

87. C. Wallis. "AIDS: A Growing Threat." *Time* 126 (August 12, 1985): 40-47.

88. _____. "A Virus As a Rosetta Stone." *Time* 12 (November 5, 1984): 91.

89. _____. "AIDS." *Newsweek* (August 12, 1985): 20-27.

90. Keven Cahill, editor. *The AIDS Epidemic*. New York: St. Martin's, 1983.

91. Planned Parenthood. *Sexually Transmitted Diseases — The Facts*. New York: Planned Parenthood, 1986.

92. Dianne Hales and Brian K. Williams. *An Invitation to Health*. 3rd ed. Menlo Park, Calif.: Benjamin-Cummings, 1986.

93. American School Health Association. *Some Questions and Answers About Gays and STDs*. 1985.

94. U.S. Department of Health and Human Services, U.S. Public Health Service. "Facts about AIDS." (July, 1983).

95. George Dintiman and Jerrold Greenberg. *Health Through Discovery*. 3rd ed. New York: Random House, 1986.

96. Wayne Payne and Dale Hahn. *Understanding Your Health*. St. Louis: C.V. Mosby, 1986.

97. Robert C. Barnes and others. *Healthy Living*. Indianapolis: Bobbs-Merrill, 1986.

98. Larry K. Olsen and others. *Health Today*. 2nd ed. New York: Macmillan, 1986.

99. Paul Insel and Walton Roth. *Core Concepts in Health*. 4th ed. Palo Alto, Calif.: Mayfield, 1986.

100. Tom Brokaw. *NBC News Special — Life, Death, and AIDS*. January 21, 1986.

101. James Curran. *AIDS — Profile of an Epidemic*. Shown on channel 12 television, Philadelphia, Pa., August 29, 1984, and updated on January 22, 1986, with Edward Asner as host.

102. Centers for Disease Control. *Morbidity and Mortality Statistics for Acquired Immune Deficiency Syndrome*. Atlanta: Centers for Disease Control, July, 1986.

103. National Center for Health Statistics. *Morbidity and Mortality Statistics for Acquired Immune Deficiency Syndrome*. Maryland: National Center for Health Statistics, July, 1986.

104. S. Weiss and others. "Screening Test for HTLV-3 Antibodies." *Journal of the American Medical Association* 253, (January 1, 1985): 221-225.

105. *The Philadelphia Inquirer*. Articles of October 30, 1985, and April 15, 1985.

106. Paul Insel and Walton Roth. *Core Concepts in Health — Update 1986*. Palo Alto, Calif.: Mayfield, 1986.

Index

adverse drug reactions 84, 186, 187
AIDS 5-27; death-rates 5, 6; definition 5; diagnosis 11-16; disease patterns 16-21; dyspnea in patients 11, 17-19; clinical manifestations 10-11; etiology 5, 8; fatality 5; history 5-6; HTLV-3 blood test 11; HTLV-3 retrovirus 5, 8; incidence 6-7; incubation period 9-10; infectious etiological agent 5, 8; Kaposi's sarcoma 19-21; laboratory pathophysiology 12-16; mode of transmission 8-9; mortality rate 5, 6; occurence 6-7; patient weakness 5, 11; period of communicability 10; pneumocystis carinii pneumonia 17-18, 22-23; population at risk 5, 7; reservoir and source of infection 8-9; social effects 26-27; suppressor cells 12-16; susceptibility and resistance 10; T-cells 12-16; treatment 21-25; vaccine research 25-26; white blood cells (WBC) in 12-16
amebiasis 40-44; definition 40; diagnosis 43; etiology 40, 41; incubation period 42; infectious etiological agent 41; mode of transmission 42; occurrence 40-41; period of communicability 42; population at risk 40, 42-43; reservoir and source of infection 41-42; signs and symptoms 43; susceptibility and resistance 42; treatment 44
amoebic dysentery *see* amebiasis
amniotic infection syndrome: in gonorrhea 71
ampicillin 87
aneurysm secondary to cardiovascular syphilis 171-172
anorectal warts 32-35

arthritis: gonococcal 67-68; Reiter's syndrome 137-139

B cells in AIDS 13, 14
biopsy: Kaposi's sarcoma 19-21; small bowel biopsy 19; chancroidal lesions 30-31; condylomata acuminata 34; granuloma inguinale lesions 98; lymphogranuloma venereum lesions 119
bladder infections: cystitis 143-147; gonorrhea 56; nonspecific non-gonococcal urethritis 123-129

candidiasis 148-152; definition 148; diagnosis 151-152; etiology 149; incubation period 150; infectious etiological agent 149; mode of transmission 149; occurrence 148; period of communicability 150; population at risk 148; reservoir and source of infection 149; signs and symptoms 151; susceptibility and resistance 150-151; treatment 152-153
cardiovascular syphilis 171-172
cerebrospinal fluid in syphilis 179
cervicitis: gonococcal 57, 80-82, 84; herpes infection 109
chancre: in syphilis 167-168
chancroid 28-31; definition 28; diagnosis 30-31; etiology 28-29; incubation period 29; infectious etiological agent 28-29; mode of transmission 29; occurrence 28; period of communicability 29; population at risk 28, 30; reservoir and source of infection 29; signs

and symptoms 30; susceptibility and resistance 30; treatment 31
Charcot's knee in syphilis 170-172
chlamydial infections: lymphogranuloma venereum 116-117; inclusion conjunctivitis 128; nonspecific nongonococcal urethritis 124-125
condom 197
condylomata acuminata 32-35; definition 32; diagnosis 34; etiology 32; incubation 33; infectious etiological agent 32; mode of transmission 33; occurrence 32; period of communicability 33; population at risk 32-33; reservoir and source of infection 33; signs and symptoms 34; susceptibility and resistance 33; treatment 34-35
condylomata lata: in syphilis 169
congenital syphilis 173-175; early 174; late 174-175
conjunctivitis: adult gonococcal 69-70, 88; gonococcal ophthalmia neonatorum 62-64, 89; inclusion conjunctivitis in NSU 128
cough: in AIDS 5, 11
crab louse infestation 130-133
cryptosporidiosis 44
cystitis 143-147
cytomegalovirus infection (CMV) 36-38; definition 36; diagnosis 38; etiology 36; incubation period 37; infectious etiological agent 36; mode of transmission 37; occurrence 36; period of communicability 37; population at risk 36, 37; reservoir and source of infection 36-37; signs and symptoms 38; susceptibility and resistance 37; treatment 38

darkfield microscopy or examination: for syphilis 176-178; for pinta 136; for yaws 195
dermatitis: gonococcal 67, 87; secondary syphilitic rash 168-169
diabetes mellitus: in candida infections 150-151
diarrhea: amebiasis 43, 44; in AIDS patients 5, 11, 19, 23; in enteric infections 39; giardiasis 46-47; shigellosis 47, 49, 50

dysuria: in gonococcal urethritis 55, 57; in herpes progenitalis 109; in nonspecific nongonococcal urethritis 126-127; in Reiter's syndrome 138- 139

educational activities for sexually transmitted diseases 201
enteric infections 39-49; amebiasis 40-44; cryptosporidiosis 44; giardiasis 44; shigellosis 47-49
epididymitis, gonococcal 56
escherichia coli infection: in nonspecific nongonococcal urethritis 124-125; in urinary tract infections 143-144
exudate discharge: in gonococcal urethritis 55, 57; in nonspecific nongonococcal urethritis 126
eye infections: adult gonococcal conjunctivitis 69-70, 88; gonococcal ophthalmia neonatorum 62-64, 89; inclusion conjunctivitis 128; Reiter's syndrome 137-138

fever: AIDS 5, 11; cytomegalovirus infection 38; enteric infections 43, 44, 46, 49; gonorrhea 57, 58, 66, 69; secondary syphilis 169
fungus infection: AIDS 11, 16; candidiasis 148-152

Gallo, Robert, M.D. 8
gardnerella vaginale vaginitis 153-155; definition 153; diagnosis 155; etiology 154; incubation period 154; infectious etiological agent 154; mode of transmission 154; occurrence 153-154; population at risk 153-154; reservoir and source of infection 154; signs and symptoms 155; susceptibility and resistance 155; treatment 155
giardiasis 44-47
gonorrhea and gonococcal disease: adult gonococcal conjunctivitis 69-71; alternative treatments 84-90; amniotic infection syndrome 71; arthritis 67-69; anaphylactic shock 84; cervicitis 57-58, 77-79, 80-83, 84-85; common names for 50;

complications 65-72; definition 50; dermatitis 67; disseminated gonococcal infection 65-72; diagnosis 72-91 (complicated gonorrhea 82-91; females 76-76; gonococcal adult conjunctivitis 88; gonococcal endocarditis 88; gonococcal infection during pregnancy 87; gonococcal meningitis 88; infant born to mother with gonorrhea 89; laboratory 80-83; males 73-76; metastatic gonorrhea 87; uncomplicated gonorrhea 84-87; vulvovaginitis 89); epidemiology 52; epididymitis 56; etiology 52-53; history 51-52; incubation period 54, 61, 63, 67, 70; infectious etiological agent 52-53; lymphadenopathy 56, 58, 59; mode of transmission 53-54; occurrence 52; ophthalmia neonatoreum 62-64; period of communicability 55; pharyngitis 59; population at risk 52, 55; proctitis 60; rectal gonorrhea 50, 60, 73, 75, 79-83, 86; reservoir and source of infection 53; salpingitis 58, 69; septicemia or gonococcemia 66-67; signs and symptoms (amniotic infection syndrome 71; cervicitis 57-58; disseminated gonococcal infection 65-66; epididymitis 56; metastatic gonorrhea 66-70; pharyngitis and tonsillitis 59; proctitis 60; urethritis 55-56; vulvovaginitis 60-62); treatment of gonorrhea 84-95; types of gonorrhea 50
granuloma inguinale 96-99; definition 96; diagnosis 98; etiology 96-97; incubation period 97; infectious etiological agent 96-97; mode of transmission 97; occurrence 96; period of communicability 97; population at risk 96, 97; reservoir and source of infection 97; signs and symptoms 97-98; susceptibility and resistance 97; treatment 98-99
Group B hemolytic streptococcal infection 100-103; definition 100; diagnosis 103; etiology 101; incubation period 102; infectious etiological agent 101; mode of transmission 102; occurrence 101; period of communicability 102; population at risk 100-101; reservoir and source of infection 101-102; signs and symptoms 102-103; susceptibility and resistance 102; treatment 103
gumma, syphilitic 171
gynecological examination: gonorrhea 77-79; syphilis 176-179; vaginitis 151-152, 155, 156, 159-161

haemophilus vaginale vaginitis *see* gardnerella vaginale vaginitis
hair loss (alopecia): in secondary syphilis 169
helper cells 12-16
hepatitis, viral 189-192; definition 189; diagnosis 192; etiology 190; incubation period 190-191; infectious etiological agent 190; mode of transmission 190; occurrence 189; period of communicability 191; population at risk 189; reservoir and source of infection 190; serum tests 192; signs and symptoms 191-192; spleenomegaly 192; susceptibility and resistance 191; treatment 192
herpes progenitalis 104-115; complications 113-115; definition 104; diagnosis 110-111; etiology 104-105; history 104; ineffective therapies 112-113; infectious etiological agent 104-105; mode of transmission 106; occurrence 104-105; period of communicability 107; population at risk 104-105; reservoir and source of infection 106; signs and symptoms 108-110; susceptibility and resistance 107-108; treatment 111-113
homosexuals, and sexually transmitted diseases 6-7; 164-165; 199

immune system: in AIDS 10, 12-16; enhancement 199-201
immunodeficiency disease: in AIDS 5, 7, 10, 12-16; in candidiasis 150-151; in condylomata acuminata 13; in urinary tract infections 146
inclusion conjunctivitis: in NSU 128
intestinal infections *see* enteric infections

Jarisch-Herxheimer reaction: in syphilis 186–187
jaundice: in hepatitis infection 191

Kaposi's sarcoma: in AIDS patients 19, 20
keratitis, interstitial, in syphilis 175

late syphilis 170–173
leukemia virus (HTLV-3) 5, 8
localized complications of gonococcal disease 65
lice, pubic 130–133
liver infection in hepatitis 192
lymphadenopathy: in AIDS 5, 11, 16; in chancroid 30; in gonorrhea 56, 58, 59; in granuloma inguinale 98; in herpes progenitalis 109–110; in lymphogranuloma venereum 118; in pinta 135; in syphilis 168–169; in yaws 194–195
lymphocytes in AIDS 12–16
lymphogranuloma venereum 116–119; definition 116; diagnosis 119; etiology 116–117; incubation period 117; infectious etiological agent 116–117; mode of transmission 117; occurrence 116; period of communicability 117; population at risk 116; reservoir and source of infection 117; signs and symptoms 118; susceptibility and resistance 117; treatment 119

meningitis: in AIDS patients 18; in herpes progenitalis 113–115; in metastatic gonorrhea 65–66; in tetriary syphilitic infection 172–173
metastatic gonorrhea 65–72
molluscum contagiosum 120–122; definition 120; diagnosis 122; etiology 120; incubation peroid 121; infectious etiological agent 120; mode of transmission 120–121; occurrence 120; period of communicability 121; population at risk 120; reservoir and source of infection 120; signs and symptoms 121; susceptibility and resistance 121; treatment 122

Montagnier, Luc, M.D. 8
Moon's or mulberry molars: in syphilitic infection 175

Neisseria gonorrhoeae 52–53
nonspecific nongonococcal urethritis 123–129; complications 128–129; definition 123; diagnosis 127; etiology 124–125; incubation period 125–126; infectious etiological agents 124–125; mode of transmission 125; occurrence 123; period of communicability 126; population at risk 123; reservoir and source of infection 125; signs and symptoms 126–127; susceptibility and resistance 126; treatment 127
nonspecific vaginitis 156
neurosyphilis 172

ophthalmia neonatorum, gonococcal 62–64
opportunistic infections: in AIDS 12–21; in candidiasis 150–151

pediculosis pubis 130–133; definition 130; diagnosis 132; etiology 130–131; incubation period 131; infectious etiological agent 130–131; mode of transmission 131; occurrence 130; period of communicability 132; population at risk 130; reservoir and source of infection 131; signs and symptoms 132; susceptibility and resistance 132; treatment 132–133
penicillin: for gonorrhea 84–94; syphilis 183–188
penicillin-resistant gonorrhea 90–95
periurethral abscess: in gonococcal urethritis 56
pharyngitis and tonsillitis: in AIDS patients 11; in gonococcal disease 59, 86; in herpes progenitalis 110; in secondary syphilis 169
pinta 134–136; definition 134; diagnosis 136; etiology 134; incubation period 135; infectious etiological agent 134; mode of transmission 134; occurrence 134; period of com-

municability 135; population at risk 134; reservoir and source of infection 134; signs and symptoms 135; susceptibility and resistance 135; treatment 136
pneumonia: in AIDS patients 5, 11, 17-18; in metastatic gonorrhea 65-66
polyarthritis: in metastatic gonorrhea 67-69; in Reiter's syndrome 138-139
pregnancy and: AIDS 9; gonorrhea 71, 87, 89; syphilis 173
prevention and control of sexually transmitted diseases 196-200
probenecid in gonorrhea treatment 84-87
proctitis, gonococcal 50, 60, 80, 81, 86

Reiter's syndrome 137-139; definition 137; diagnosis 139; etiology 137; incubation period 138; infectious etiological agent 137; mode of transmission 137; occurrence 137; period of communicability 138; population at risk 137; reservoir and source of infection 137; signs and symptoms 138-139; susceptibility and resistance 138; treatment 139
risk factors: AIDS 7; reduction of risk factors for STD's 196-200

salpingitis, gonococcal 69, 78, 85-86
scabies 140-142; definition 140; diagnosis 142; etiology 140; incubation period 141; infectious etiological agent 140; mode of transmission 141; occurrence 140; period of communicability 141; population at risk 140; reservoir and source of infection 140; signs and symptoms 141; susceptibility and resistance 141; treatment 142
secondary syphilitic infection 168-169
septicemia, gonococcal 66-67, 87-88
shigellosis 47-50; definition 47; diagnosis 50; etiology 47-48; incubation period 48; infectious etiological agent 47-48; mode of transmission 48; occurrence 47; period of communicability 48; population at risk 47, 48; reservoir and source of infection 48; signs and symptoms 48; susceptibility and resistance 48-49; treatment 50
syphilis, venereal 162-188; alternative treatments 184-188; anaphylactic shock 187; Charcot's knee 170-172; congenital syphilis 173-175; definition 162; diagnosis 175-183; epidemiology 167; etiology 165; history 162-164; incubation period 166; infectious etiological agent 165; latent syphilis 169-170; mode of transmission 165-166; occurrence 164-165; period of communicability 166-167; population at risk 164-165; primary syphilitic infection 167-168; reservoir and source of infection 165; secondary syphilitic infection 168-169; serological tests 177-179; signs and symptoms of syphilis 167-175; spinal fluid examination 179; susceptibility and resistance 167; tertiary syphilitic infection 170-172; treatment 183-188

tabes dorsalis: in tertiary syphilis 172
tetracycline hydrocholoride: dangers in pregnancy 93; in gonorrhea 84-87, 90, 92, 93; in nonspecific nongonococcal urethritis 127; in syphilis 184
thrush: in AIDS patients 5, 11, 16; in candidiasis 151
tonsillitis and pharyngitis: in AIDS patients 11; in gonococcal pharyngitis 59, 80, 81, 86; in herpes progenitalis 110
treponema pallidum: in syphilitic infection 165
trichomoniasis 156-161; definition 156; diagnosis 159-161; etiology 157; incubation period 158; infectious etiological agent 157; mode of transmission 158; occurrence 156-157; period of communicability 158; population at risk 156-157; reservoir and source of infection 157-158; signs and symptoms 159; susceptibility and resistance 158; treatment 161

ulcers, chancroidal 30
urethritis: in gonorrhea 55–57; in herpes progenitalis 109–110; nonspecific nongonococcal 126; in Reiter's syndrome 138–139; in urinary tract infections 143–147
urination: frequency (in gonococcal urethritis) 55–57; frequency (in nonspecific nongonococcal urethritis) 126; difficulty (in nonspecific nongonococcal urethritis) 126; and pain *see* dysuria
urinary tract infections 143–147; definition 143; diagnosis 147; etiology 143–144; incubation period 145; infectious etiological agent 143–144; mode of transmission 145; occurrence 143; period of communicability 145; population at risk 143; reservoir and source of infection 145; signs and symptoms 146; susceptibility and resistance 146; treatment 147
urine: bloody in gonorrhea 56; difficult passage of in NSU 126
urine culture and sensitivity: in gonorrhea 80–81; in nonspecific nongonococcal urethritis 147

vaccine research: in AIDS 25–26; in gonorrhea 55; in herpes progenitalis 112
vaginal discharge: in candidiasis 151; in gardnerella vaginale vaginitis 155; in gonococcal cervicitis 57–58; in nonspecific vaginitis 156; in trichomoniasis 159
vaginitis 148–161; candidiasis 148–152; gardnerella vaginale 153–155; nonspecific 156; trichomoniasis 156–161; vulvovaginitis, gonococcal 50, 60–62, 89–90
viral forms of sexually transmitted diseases: AIDS 5, 8; condylomata acuminata 32–35; cytomegalovirus infections 36–38; hepatitis 189–192; herpes progenitalis 104–115
vulvovaginitis: in gonorrhea 50, 60–62, 89–90

warts, genital 32–35

yeast infections: in AIDS patients 5, 11, 16; in candidiasis 149
yaws 193–195; definition 193; diagnosis 195; etiology 193; incubation period 194; infectious etiological agent 193; mode of transmission 194; occurrence 193; period of communicability 194; population at risk 193; reservoir and source of infection 193; signs and symptoms 194–195; susceptibility and resistance 194; treatment 195